SpeakEasy Spanish™

MW00342404

SURVIVAL SPANISH
FOR
PHARMACISTS

Myelita Melton, MA

SpeakEasy Communications, Incorporated

SpeakEasy's Survival Spanish for Pharmacists

Author: Myelita A. Melton
Cover Design: Ellen Wass Beckerman
Published by SpeakEasy Communications, Incorporated
116 Sea Trail Drive
Mooresville, NC 28117-8493
USA

ISBN   0-9786998-3-1
ISBN: 13: 978-0-9786998-3-3

Survival Spanish for Pharmacists, SpeakEasy Spanish, SpeakEasy's Survival Spanish, SpeakEasy's Survival Spanish for Healthcare, and SpeakEasySpanish.com are either trademarks or registered trademarks of SpeakEasy Communications, Inc. in the United States and/or other countries.

The content of this book is furnished for informational use only, is subject to change without notice, and should not be construed as a commitment by SpeakEasy Communications, Incorporated. SpeakEasy Communications, Incorporated assumes no responsibility or liability for any errors, omissions, or inaccuracies that may appear in the informational content contained in this guide.

Survival Spanish for Pharmacists
Table of Contents

Using This Material

SpeakEasy's Survival Spanish for Pharmacists. is designed for adults with no previous experience in the Spanish language. Through research and interviews with professionals in your field, we have developed this material to be a practical guide to using Spanish on the job. Wherever possible, we use the similarities between English and Spanish to facilitate your success.

Throughout the manual you will find study tips and pronunciation guides that will help you to say the words correctly. In the guides, we have broken down the Spanish words for you by syllables, choosing English words that closely approximate the Spanish sound needed. This method makes learning Spanish more accessible because it doesn't seem so foreign. When you see letters that are **BOLD** in the guide, say that part of the word the loudest. The bold capital letters are there to show you where the emphasis falls in that word.

At SpeakEasy Communications, we believe that *communication* is more important than *conjugation*, and that what you learn must be practical for what you do. We urge you to set realistic, practical goals. Make practice a regular part of your day and you will be surprised at the progress you make!

SpeakEasy's Secrets to Learning Spanish

Congratulations on your decision to learn Spanish! This decision is one of the smartest choices you will ever make considering the increasing diversity in our country. It's definitely one you will never regret. You are now among a growing number of America's visionary leaders, who want to build more trusting relationships with Hispanic-Americans, the fastest growing segment of our population.

Learning Spanish is going to open many doors for you, and it will affect you in ways you can't imagine. By learning Spanish, you will be able to work more efficiently and safely in almost every workplace in the nation. Since bilingual employees are currently in short supply nationwide, you will find increasing job opportunities in almost every profession. In addition, you will be able to build stronger relationships with Latinos you meet anywhere you go. There's also another added benefit: You are going to raise your communication skills to a whole new level.

As an adult, learning a new language requires a certain mind set. It takes time, patience and more than a little stubbornness. Think about it. You didn't learn English overnight. You began crying as an infant. That was your first attempt at communication. Later you uttered syllables. When you did, your parents thought you were the world's smartest child, and they rewarded you constantly. After a few years you began to make simple sentences. By the time you reached your first class in school, if you were like me, you couldn't stop talking. So, you can't expect to know everything about Spanish by studying it for only a few weeks. You must give Spanish some time to sink in just as English did.

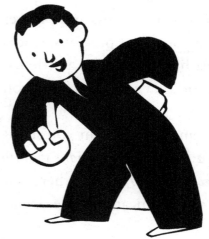

It's also important for you to realize that adults learn languages differently than children do. Kids learn by listening and by imitating. For them, learning Spanish or any other second language is relatively easy, because their brains are learning naturally. It's part of human development. Then we reach puberty and everything changes! Your body sets your speech pattern for its native language. For many people, this is the age when their language learning center slows down or turns completely off. Your body just figures it doesn't need it anymore. Coincidentally, this slow-down occurs about the time that you hit your seventh grade Spanish class. That's why learning Spanish seemed to be so hard — that, and the huge amount of very impractical things you were forced to learn. As a result of this physical change in puberty, adults tend to learn languages more visually. Listening and imitating are still important; especially when paired with a visual cue. Most adults benefit from seeing a Spanish word spelled phonetically and hearing it at the same time. This combination helps your brain make sense of the new sounds.

Adults are also practical learners. If you see a reason for what you are learning, you will find it easier to accomplish. It is very true that if you practice your Spanish daily, you are less likely to lose it.! You are *never* too old to learn Spanish.

If you did take Spanish in high school or college, you are going to be pleasantly surprised when words and phrases you thought you had forgotten begin to come back to you. That previous experience with other languages is still in your mind. It's just hidden away in a little-used filing cabinet. Soon that cabinet will open up again and that's going to help you learn new words even faster.

Here's another thought you should consider. *What they told you in the traditional foreign language classroom was not exactly correct.* There's no such thing as *"perfect Spanish"* just as there is no *"perfect English."* This fact leaves the door for good communication wide open!

The secret to learning Spanish is having *self-confidence and a great sense of humor.* To build self-confidence, you must realize that the entire learning experience is painless and fun. Naturally, you are going to make mistakes: everyone does. We all make mistakes in English too! So get ready to laugh and learn. *Don't believe that you have to have a perfect Spanish sentence in your head before you say something.*

It's very important for you to say what you know— even if it's only a word or two. The point is to communicate. Communication doesn't have to be "pretty" or perfect to be effective.

Español is one of the world's most precise and expressive languages. Consider these other important facts as you begin to "*habla español*":

- ✓ English and Spanish share a common Latin heritage, so literally thousands of words in our two languages are either *similar* or *identical.*

- ✓ Your ability to communicate is the most important thing, so your grammar and pronunciation don't have to be "*perfect*" for people to understand you.

- ✓ Many practical and common expressions in Spanish can be communicated with a few simple words.

- ✓ As the number of Latinos in the United States increases, your opportunities to practice increase. Saying even a phrase or two in Spanish every day will help you learn faster.

- ✓ Relax! People who enjoy their learning experiences acquire Spanish at a much faster pace than others.

- ✓ Set realistic goals and establish reasonable practice habits.

- ✓ When you speak even a little Spanish, you are showing a respect for the Hispanic culture and its people.

- ✓ Even a little Spanish or *poco español* goes a long way!

As you begin the process of learning Spanish, you are going to notice a few important differences. Speaking Spanish is going to feel and sound a little odd to you at first. This feeling is completely normal because you are using muscles in your face that English doesn't require, and your inner ear is not accustomed to hearing you speak Spanish. People tell me it sounds and feels like a cartoon character has gotten inside your head! Don't let that stop you. Just keep right on going!

Many Americans know more Spanish than they realize and they can pronounce many words perfectly. Review the list below. How many of the Spanish words in it, do you recognize? Using what you already know about Spanish will enable you to learn new things easier and faster — it's a great way to build your confidence.

Amigos Similares y Familiares

Americano	Amigo	Hospital	Español	Doctor
Loco	Hotel	Oficina	Agua	Fiesta
Dinero	Señor	Señorita	Señora	Sombrero
Burrito	Taco	Olé	No problema	Accidente
Nachos	Salsa	Grande	Quesadilla	Margarita
Aspirina	Medicina	Cerveza	Hospital	Emergencia

The Sounds of Spanish

No se preocupe. Don't worry. One of your biggest concerns about speaking a new language will be speaking it well enough so that others can understand you. Spanish is close enough to English that making mistakes along the way won't hurt your ability to communicate.

The most important sounds in Spanish consist of *five* vowels. Each one is pronounced the way it is written. Spanish vowels are never *silent*. Even when there are two vowels together in a word, both of them will stand up and be heard.

A	(ah)	as in mama
E	(eh)	as in "hay or the "eh" in set
I	(ee)	as in deep
O	(oh)	as in open
U	(oo)	as in spoon

4

Here are the other sounds you'll need to remember. Always pronounce them the same way. Spanish is a very consistent language. The sounds the letters make don't shift around as much as they do in English.

Spanish Letter		**English Sound**
C	(before an e or i)	s as in Sam: **cero**: SAY-row
G	(before an e or i)	h as in he: **energía**: n-air-HE-ah
		emergencia: a-mare-HEN-see-ah
H		silent: **hacienda**: ah-see-N-da
J		h as in hot: **Julio**, HOO-lee-oh
LL		y as in yoyo: **tortilla**, tor- TEE-ya
Ñ		ny as in canyon: **español**, es-pan- NYOL
QU		k as in kit: **tequila**, tay-KEY-la
RR		Trilled r sound: **burro**, BOO-row
V		v as in Victor: **Victor**, Vic-TOR
Z		s as in son: **Gonzales**, gone-SA-les

The Other Consonants: The remaining letters in Spanish have very similar sounds to their equivalents in English.

**Note: People from Latin American countries have a variety of accents just like Americans do. In certain areas of Latin America people tend to pronounce the letter "v" more like the English letter "b." This tendency is particularly true in parts of Mexico. In other Latin American countries a "v" sounds like an English "v." If you learned to switch the "v" sound for a "b" sound in high school or college Spanish classes, don't change your habit; however, if you haven't had any experience with Spanish before now, don't sweat the small stuff! Pronounce the "v" as you normally would.

The Spanish Alphabet
El alfabeto español

A	ah	**J**	HO-ta	**R**	AIR-ray
B	bay	**K**	ka	**RR**	EH-rray
C	say	**L**	L-ay	**S**	S-ay
CH	chay	**LL**	A-yea	**T**	tay
D	day	**M**	M-ay	**U**	oo
E	A or EH	**N**	N-ay	**V**	vay
F	f-AY	**Ñ**	N-yea	**W**	DOE-blay-vay
G	hay	**O**	oh	**X**	A-kees
H	AH-chay	**P**	pay	**Y**	ee-gree-A-gah
I	ee	**Q**	coo	**Z**	SAY-ta

Did you notice something different about the Spanish alphabet? It has four letters the English alphabet doesn't have. Can you find them?

The Four "Extra" Letters

Look carefully at the table above which contains the Spanish alphabet. Did you notice that the Spanish language has more letters in its alphabet than English does? There are thirty letters in the Spanish alphabet. Even though Spanish has more letters in its alphabet, none of them will present *problemas* for you. Here are the four extra letters and words in which they are used:

CH   Sounds like the following English words: Charlie and chocolate. **Example:** Nacho and macho

LL   Sounds essentially like an English "y," however, you will hear slight variations depending on where the person is from who is speaking Spanish with you. **Example:** Tortilla (tor-T-ya)

Ñ   Sounds like a combination of "ny" as in canyon or onion: **Example:** español (es-pan-**NYOL**)

RR   This letter is a "trilled" sound. Practice by taking your tongue and placing it in the roof of your mouth just behind your front teeth. Now blow air across the tip of your tongue and make it flutter.

    This sound can be difficult for some adults to make. It's only strange because you are moving your tongue muscle in a new way. Since there are no words in English with trilled sounds, you just never learned to move your tongue that way. Children learning Spanish have no trouble with this sound at all. Like any new activity, it will take time, patience and practice! Don't let a problem with the trilled "r" stop you from speaking. Essentially the sounds of the English "r" and the Spanish "r" are the same. To start with, say the double "r" a bit louder than a single "r." **Example:** Burrito (boo-**REE**-toe)

The Spanish Accent

There are two types of accent marks in Spanish. Both marks are important and do different things. One of the marks called a "tilde." It is only found over the letter "N." The accent mark over Ñ makes it into a different letter entirely. It's one of four letters in the Spanish alphabet that the English alphabet doesn't have. The Ñ changes the sound of the letter to a combination of "ny." You'll hear the sound that this important letter makes in the English words "canyon" and "onion."

Occasionally you will see another accent mark over a letter in a Spanish word. The accent mark or "slash" mark shows you where to place vocal emphasis. When you see an accent mark over a letter in a Spanish word, say that part of the word louder. We indicate these accented syllables in our pronunciation guides with bold, capital letters. **Example:** José (ho-**SAY**)

Pronouncing Spanish Words

The pronunciation of Spanish words follows basic, consistent rules. This regular pattern makes it easier to learn. Here are some points to remember:

1. Most Spanish words that end with vowels are stressed or emphasized on the *next to the last* syllable.

   Señorita: sen-your-**REE**-ta   Jalapeño: ha-la-**PAIN**-yo

2. Look for an accent mark. If the Spanish word has an accent in it, that's the emphasized syllable.

   José: ho-**SAY**   ¿Cómo está?: **KO**-mo es-**TA**

3. Words that end in consonants are stressed on the *final* syllable.

   Doctor: doc-**TOR**   Hotel: oh-**TELL**

Spanish Punctuation Marks

Spanish has two different punctuation marks than English does. Both of them are upside down versions of English punctuation marks. They signal that something other than a simple declarative sentence is just ahead.

First, there's the upside down question mark (¿). You will see it at the beginning of all questions. It's there to let you know that what follows is a question, so you know in advance to give your voice an upward inflection. It's the same inflection we use in English.

   Example: Do you speak English?   ¿Habla inglés?

Second, there's the upside down exclamation mark (¡). It lets you know that what follows should be vocally emphasized. **Example:** Hi!   ¡Hola!

Spanglish

Much of the southwestern part of the United States originally belonged to Mexico. In 1848, after the US-Mexican War, the US border moved south to the Rio Grande River. The treaty that was signed at the end of the conflict transformed Spanish-speaking Mexicans into Americans overnight! Imagine waking up one morning and finding out that you are a citizen of another country—and that you have to learn a new language! As a result, an entirely new slang language was born that mixes the best of both worlds: *Spanglish*. This language has been growing and evolving ever since.

In America, Spanglish really began to come into its own in the early 1970s. At that time it gained popularity and vocabulary. Now, people who use Spanglish span generations, classes, and nationalities. It's heard in pop music, seen in print, and used in conversations throughout Latin America.

Spanglish isn't just an American phenomenon. Immigrants may turn to Spanglish out of necessity while they are learning English, and bilingual speakers use it because it's convenient. If you listen to native speakers carefully, you will hear them use a mixture of languages. Sometimes in the middle of a conversation, you may hear an English word or two. People who speak Spanish tend to use whatever word or phrase suits their purpose and is most descriptive. In general conversation it doesn't matter what language it is. Even though Spanglish is still frowned upon in most traditional language classrooms, it really is a great tool for many people.

What Spanglish words have you heard? Before automatically deciding that a word is Spanglish, you should look it up in a Spanish-English dictionary. You might be surprised when you find the word you thought was Spanglish is actually one of the many "friendly" words or cognates between our languages. The list on the following page contains many "amigos familiares" for you to practice.

More Amigos Familiares

Using what you've learned about how Spanish sounds, practice the words listed below. Each word bears a strong resemblance to its English counterpart or is a common Spanish word many people use who doesn't speak Spanish. Begin by carefully and slowly pronouncing each word on the list. If you are having trouble, go back and review the vowel sounds again.

Absceso	Epidermis	Nutrición
Accidente	Espina	Ovario
Aeropuerto	Estómago	Paciente
Apartamento	Familia	Penicilina
Aplicación	Fémur	Persona
Baño	Fiebre	Plato
Bebé	Ginecólogo	Policía
Cápsula	Hemorroides	Posible
Cardíaco	Hospital	Progreso
Cartílago	Identificación	Rápido
Caución	Infección	Recto
Chocolate	Inhalador	Remedio
Cirugía	Inflamación	Respiración
Cortisona	Intestino	Síndrome
Colesterol	Loción	Supervisor
Depresión	Macarrones	Supositorio
Dieta	Medicina	Tableta
Doctor	Minuto	Televisión
Epidermis	Momento	Tratamiento
Emergencia	Monitor	Úlcera

Muchos Ways to "Practicar"

The more you listen to and use your *español,* the easier it will be for you to learn it. There are lots of creative ways to practice that won't cost you any money. Try these super techniques for improving your skills:

- ✓ Next time you're at a Mexican restaurant, order your food in *español.*

- ✓ Start slowly. Practice one sound each week.

- ✓ Read Spanish language newspapers. They are usually free and easily available.

- ✓ Listen to Spanish language radio stations.

- ✓ Watch Spanish language television.

- ✓ Rent Spanish language videos; especially cartoons.

- ✓ Buy Spanish CDs and listen to them in the car while you commute.

- ✓ And—speaking of CDs, there is such a variety of Latin *música* available, something will be right for you. Listening to music is a great way to train your ears to Spanish and have fun doing it. Personally, I like anything by Carlos Santana or Marc Anthony. Who do you like?

- ✓ Visit Internet sites like *www.about.com* or *www.studyspanish.com.* You can find all kinds of information there about the Spanish language. They have a wonderful, free newsletter that comes to you via e-mail. Most search engines have some sort of Spanish section. An on-line search will turn up lots of treasures!

- ✓ Next time you listen to a baseball game, keep track of all the Hispanic names you hear.

- ✓ Speak Spanish every time the opportunity presents itself. Practice is the only way to get over your nervousness.

- ✓ Try to learn with a friend at work and practice together.

Tips and Techniques for Comunicación

It's important to remember, when you're trying to communicate with a person who is "limited in English proficiency," *patience is a virtue*! Put yourself in their shoes and think how you would feel if the roles were reversed. Here are some easy things you can do to make the conversation easier for both of you.

✓ Speak slowly and distinctly.

✓ Do not use slang expressions or colorful terms.

✓ Get straight to the point! Unnecessary words cloud your meaning.

✓ Speak in a normal tone. Speaking *loudly* doesn't help anyone understand you any better!

✓ Look for cues to meaning in body language and facial expressions. Use gestures of your own to get your point across.

✓ You may not receive good eye contact. Do not interpret the lack of eye contact negatively.

✓ Latinos tend to stand closer to each other than North Americans do when they talk with each other, so your personal space could feel crowded. Stand your ground!

✓ Feel free to use gestures and body language of your own to communicate.

✓ Because of the way languages are learned, it is likely that the person you are talking to understands more of what you are saying than he is able to verbalize. *So, be careful what you say!* No matter what the language, we always understand the bad words first!

TIPS & TIDBITS
Throughout your book look for the light bulb you see above. This section will give you helpful hints and cultural information designed to help you learn Spanish more easily.

Beginning Words & Phrases

In no time you will start gaining confidence. Your Latino patients and colleagues will be delighted you are learning to speak *español*. Simple words like please and thank you show respect and courtesy. That will help you to establish rapport.

English	Español	Guide
Hi!	¡Hola!	**OH**-la
How are you?	¿Cómo está?	**CO**-mo es-**TA**
Fine	Muy bien.	mooy b-**N**
So so	Así así	ah-**SEE** ah-**SEE**
Bad	Mal	mal
Good morning	Buenos días	boo-**WAY**-nos **DEE**-ahs
Good afternoon	Buenas tardes	boo-**WAY**-nas **TAR**-days
Good night	Buenas noches.	boo-**WAY**-nas **NO**-chase
Sir or Mister	Señor	sen-**YOUR**
Mrs. or Ma'am	Señora	sen-**YOUR**-ah
Miss	Señorita	sen-your-**REE**-ta
What's your name?	¿Cómo se llama?	**CO**-mo say **YA**-ma
My name is ____.	Me llamo ____.	may **YA**-mo
Nice to meet you.	¡Mucho gusto!	**MOO**-cho **GOO**-stow
Thank you.	Gracias.	**GRA**-see-ahs
Please!	¡Por favor!	pour-fa-**VOR**
You're welcome. The pleasure is mine.	De nada. El gusto es mío.	day **NA** da el **GOO**-stow es **ME**-oh
I'm sorry.	Lo siento.	low-see-**N**-toe
Excuse me.	¡Perdón!	pear-**DON**
Good-bye	Adiós	ah-dee-**OS**

Spanish Sounds Rápido — What Do I Do Now?

Be honest! One of the reasons you are hesitant to speak Spanish is that it sounds so fast! Naturally, you're afraid you won't understand. Here are some phrases that will help you; make learning them a priority. *¿Comprende, amigo?*

English	Español	Guide
I don't understand.	No comprendo.	no com-**PREN**-doe
Do you understand?	¿Comprende?	com-**PREN**-day
I speak a little Spanish.	Hablo poco español.	**AH**-blow **POE**-co es-pan-**NYOL**
Do you speak English?	¿Habla inglés?	**AH**-bla eng-**LACE**
Repeat, please.	Repita, por favor.	ray-**PETE**-ah pour fa-**VOR**
I'm studying Spanish.	Estudio español.	es-**TOO**-d-oh es-pan-**NYOL**
Write it, please	Escribe, por favor.	es-**SCREE**-bay pour fa-**VOR**
Speak more slowly, please.	Habla más despacio, por favor.	**AH**-bla mas des-**PA**-see-oh pour fa-**VOR**
Thanks for your patience.	Gracias por su paciencia.	**GRA**-see-ahs pour sue pa-see-**N**-see-ah
How do you say it in Spanish?	¿Cómo se dice en español?	**CO**-mo say **DEE**-say n es-pan-**NYOL**
Where are you from?	¿De dónde es?	day **DON**-day es
May I help you?	¿Puedo ayudarle?	pooh-**A**-doe eye-you-**DAR**-lay

The key is <u>not</u> to pánico.

Your Spanish-speaking employee or friend is having just as much trouble understanding you, as you are having understanding him! Hang in there! Between the two of you, **comunicación** will begin to take place.

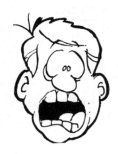

Conversaciones

Test Yourself: Using the vocabulary on pages 14-15, how would you say these phrases in español

Practice Conversation I

Sr. García: Good morning. How are you?

Usted: Fine, thanks, and you?

Sr. García: Fine, thank you.

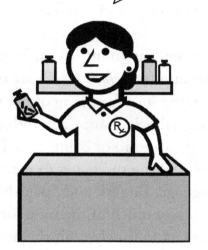

¡Hola!
Soy la
farmacéutica

Practice Conversation II

Usted My name is . I speak a little Spanish. What's your name?

Sra. García: My name is Carla García Hernandez.

I speak a little English.

Usted Nice to meet you.

Sra. García Yes, nice to meet you.

The Emergency Conversation

Good morning or hi

My name is .

I speak a little Spanish.

Do you speak English?

Speak more slowly, please.

Thank you.

Why Does Spanish Sound So Fast?

To people who speak English as their native language, the Spanish language sounds extremely fast. There are several reasons for this astute observation. First, Spanish flows from one word to another without an obvious pause between words. Sometimes it appears that native speakers only pause when they need to breathe! As a result of this gliding from word to word, it's difficult for many beginners to distinguish where one word starts and another word stops. This fact alone is a great reason to put the phrase "speak more slowly please" (*Habla más despacio, por favor.*) at the top of your "to learn" list. By using this phrase, the person you are talking to will become more conscious of their verbal speed. They will say words more slowly, and you'll begin to hear the words more distinctly.

Another important reason Spanish why sounds like a star ship at warp speed is that pronouns (*see chart p. 17*) are often omitted. Why? People who speak Spanish are listening for the ending of the verb in the sentence to tell them who or what is being talked about. Each verb ending is different, so it's easy for them to tell who is being talked to or being talked about. Native speakers of the Spanish language aren't taking their cues to meaning from pronouns at all. In this aspect of language, English and Spanish are very different. Since the pronouns aren't necessary much of the time for precise communication in Spanish, many native speakers routinely omit them.

When you compare how basic verbs sound in English and Spanish, you will realize that many regular English verbs in the present tense sound exactly the alike. Here's a good example: I speak, you speak, we speak, they speak, etc. If it weren't for the pronoun at the beginning of the sentence, we wouldn't know what or who was being talked about at all because the verbs are identical! Since many of the verbs forms sound the same, people who speak English are listening for the pronoun at the beginning of the sentence to tell them what's being discussed.

If you have studied Spanish previously, you might have learned how to ask this basic question "how are you" as *¿Cómo está <u>usted</u>?* This form includes the pronoun "*usted.*" It's important to realize you may not hear it said that way in the "real world." Both *¿Cómo está usted?* and *¿Cómo está?* mean exactly the same thing. One form isn't better than the other or more polite. So, it's fine to drop most pronouns.

In fact, when you do drop them, you begin to sound more natural, and as an added bonus, you'll make fewer mistakes!

English	Español	Guide
I	Yo	yo
You (informal)	Tú	too
He	Él	L
She	Ella	A-ya
You (Polite)	Usted	oo-**STED**
We	Nosotros	no-**SO**-tros
	Nosotras *(f)*	no-**SO**-tras
They	Ellos	A-yos
	Ellas *(f)*	A-yas
You (Plural)	Ustedes	oo-**STED**-es

TIPS & TECHNIQUES

If you learned Spanish in high school, what you studied was possibly Castilian Spanish. That is the form of Spanish which is spoken in Spain. That type of Spanish has several different features from the language as it is spoken in Latin America. One of the unique features of Castilian Spanish is the use of the word *vosotros (-as)* or the polite form of "you." In Latin America, this form is not used. The pronoun *usted* is used instead. In this book we are concentrating on Latin American Spanish because that's what you are most likely to hear and use.

Which "You" Are You?
Tú or Usted

Review the table of pronouns on the preceding page. Did you notice that there are many different ways to say "you"? The pronoun *"you"* is one of the most important ones on the entire list. You will use it often, and when you do, you will have several decisions to make.

First, there is the choice of using either the Castilian or Latin American forms: *vosotros* or *usted*. We've already decided to go with Latin American Spanish since it's what you are most likely to hear in the workplace.

Next, we must decide whether it's best to be informal or more polite when we address patients and their families. On the job which should you choose *tú* or *usted*? If you studied Spanish in high school or college, you might be more comfortable using *tú*.

In your classroom setting where you and your friends were the same age and on a first name basis, tú was correct. Because you used it so much in school, it might be the word that comes into your mind first now.

Now your needs are different and your situation has changed. In SpeakEasy Spanish™ we emphasize the need for courtesy in every phrase and form we present. Spanish is a language that is designed to show ultimate courtesy and respect, so let's use that to our advantage. In the workplace with adults *usted* is the correct form of address to use.

Many Latin Americans, especially older ones, are uncomfortable with using a professional's first name quickly. For Spanish-speaking adults to move from addressing each other with *usted* to the use of *tú*, a long-term relationship must be established. Later on when you begin to work with verbs, you will also see the verb form which matches *usted* is simpler to use. By using *usted*, you can't go wrong. You'll be showing courtesy and respect to your patients, and decreasing your chances of making errors in your verbs. *¡Fantástico!*

Spanish Nouns
Can words really have a gender?

¡Sí! Spanish belongs to the "romance" language family. Calling Spanish a "romance" language doesn't mean that it has anything to do with love. Where Spanish is concerned, it's all about the ancient Romans. Like many European languages, Spanish is an offshoot of Latin. Classification of nouns into groups or categories remains a common feature of each language in the romance language group today.

In ancient times, people had even more challenges learning another language than we do today. There were no tapes, CDs, or internet and few foreign language teachers. For that matter, there weren't many schools either! Most folks simply learned other languages through time consuming trial and error.

To help the challenging process along, words were placed into categories based upon how they sounded. This process organized the material and made words easier to learn. These categories were often described as "masculine," "feminine," or even "neuter." From these descriptions, people began talking about words in terms of their gender. Even though the word "gender" is misleading, the tendency to group words by sound helped people learn more quickly.

Because Spanish evolved from Latin, it has maintained two category divisions for centuries. The categories are called masculine and feminine. Even though Spanish can and will evolve as all languages do, the concept of "gender" categories in español is not likely to change.

Here are the most important points to remember about nouns and their "categories":

1. Usually, words are grouped by how they sound, not by what they mean. There will always be a few exceptions!

2. Languages are a lot like the people who use them: They don't always follow the rules!

19

3. If the Spanish noun is referring to a person, the letter will often indicate the sex of that individual. For example: a doctor, who is a man, is a "doctor" A woman, who is a doctor, is a "doctora."

4. Words in the "masculine" category usually end with the letter "O".

5. Words in the "feminine" category usually end with the letter "A".

6. El, la, los and las are very important words. They all mean "the". They are the clues you need to tell you a word's category.

Articles: Making Connections

The words in Spanish that mark which category a noun falls into are some of the most commonly used words in the entire Spanish language. These words are called "articles." In English these are the words the, a, or an. You'll not only hear them often in Spanish, you'll use them often too.

Nouns and their articles match each other like identical twins. Here's how it works. Match the category of article and noun as either masculine or feminine. Then, determine if the noun you are using is singular or plural.

Even though the correct use of articles is an important feature of Spanish, nothing is more important than the noun! If you are unsure about which article to use, simply leave it out. The noun you say carries all the meaning. In the grand scheme of things, this mistake is relatively minor.

It's much more important to say the word that carries the meaning than the word that indicates category and number. Eliminating the article on occasion or using the wrong one won't prevent you from being understood. You might not be perfect in your grammar usage, but you will be effective in your communications. Always remember:

Everyone makes mistakes—even native speakers!

Definite and Indefinite Articles

English	Español	Guide
The (singular)	*El (m) La (f)	L la
The (plural)	Los Las	los las
A or an	Un (m) Una (f)	oon OO-na
Some (plural)	Unos Unas	OO-nos OO-nahs

A Word about Adjectives

Describing things in Spanish can present problems for English speakers. There are several reasons why using adjectives may give us trouble.

First, there is the position of the adjective in relation to the noun. In English, descriptive words go in front of the noun like "white cat," for example. In Spanish, the noun is the most important element, so it comes first. White cat is *gato blanco*. It is the opposite of our word order. However, it gets more complicated because there are a few basic adjectives which show size or quantity that are placed in front of the noun, just as in English. These include words like large (*grande*) and small (*pequeño*), along with numbers.

For example: a large white cat is *un grande gato blanco*.

Second, since Spanish nouns are divided into masculine and feminine categories, the adjective must match its noun by category. This means that from time to time you will need to match the letter at the end of the adjective and make it the same letter that is at the end of the noun.

You must also match the adjective to the noun by number (singular or plural). This matching sound feature of Spanish is one of the main reasons it has such a musical sound.

Example:

One large white cat	Uno grande gato blanco
Three large white cats	Tres grandes gatos blancos
One large white house	Una grande casa blanca
Six large white houses	Seis grandes casas blancas

Adding Description with Adjectives

These common adjectives are shown as you would find them in a Spanish dictionary. Usually the masculine form of the word is what you find in the dictionary. Often you will see (a) written after the word to indicate the feminine form.

As indicated in the table below, use the adjectives without changing their ending when you pair them with singular words in the masculine category. You will place most of these adjectives behind the noun instead of in front of it.

Change the "o" at the end of the adjective to an "a" if you need it to match a word which is feminine in category.

If the adjective ends with the letter "e," you won't need to change anything to make it feminine! Also, don't forget to add an "s" at the end of your adjective to match it with plural words.

**Note: Position adjectives which indicate a quantity, number or size in front of the noun instead of behind it.

Common Adjectives

English	Español	Guide
Good	Bueno	boo-**WAY**-no
Bad	Mal	mal
Big	Grande	**GRAN**-day
Little	Pequeño	pay-**CANE**-yo
More	Más	mas
Less	Menos	**MAY**-nos
Hot	Caliente	ca-lee-**N**-tay
Cold	Frío	**FREE**-oh
Sick	Enfermo	n-**FAIR**-mo

Yours, Mine or Ours

Where is **your** son? **My** son is in high school. Notice the words in bold face type. Each of them is a possessive adjective. Now that you understand the basics about adjectives and their relationship to nouns in Spanish, let's move on to adjectives which indicate possession. They may be the easiest for you to learn and use correctly immediately.

Possessive adjectives are easy to use in Spanish for two basic reasons.

1. They come in front of the noun like they do in English.
2. Possessive adjectives do not show the gender or category of the noun they are paired with.

These common adjectives only show that the noun they are paired with is singular or plural. That makes them not only easy to use, but practical to use as well.

English	Español		Guide
My	Mi		me
	Mis		meese
Your	Tu		too
	Tus		toos
His, her or Your (polite)	Su		sue
	Sus		seus
Our	Nuestro (-os)		new-ES-tro
	Nuestra (-as)		new-ES-tra

TIPS & TECHNIQUES

Celebrate Hispanic Heritage Month and Día de la Raza in October. It's more inclusive to celebrate Hispanic heritage at that time because it recognizes the diversity among Latinos and doesn't highlight just one country. Having a fiesta during Hispanic Heritage month is much better than a "Cinco de mayo" celebration because it is only observed in Mexico. Celebrating it could alienate your Latino patients from other countries.

Using Adjectives to Differentiate

Adjectives are the great character actors of the language stage. They play many vital roles by putting on different faces and costumes to give us a variety of linguistic details. They certainly spice up our speech! Along with nouns and verbs, adjectives provide a powerful foundation for basic conversation.

The primary function of any adjective is to describe, but they often do much more than that. Adjectives can indicate whether an object belongs to us or someone else, and they can also be used to point out or differentiate one object from another.

For example, you'll use this set of adjectives to say "**this** report is good" or "**that** grade could be better." Demonstrative adjectives make a practical addition to your growing vocabulary, and they are easy to use.

Demonstrative adjectives, like other adjectives in Spanish, are paired with a noun according to its gender or category and its plurality. Note that the feminine forms of these adjectives all have the letter "a" near the end of the word. That's a good indicator that you will pair it with a noun that's feminine in category.

The plural forms of demonstrative adjectives end with the letter "s." Use them when you are pointing out more than one thing.

Where location is concerned, place your demonstrative adjective directly before the noun. It takes the same spot in front of the noun just as it does in English.

Point It Out: Using Adjectives to Demonstrate

English	Español	Guide
This	Este	ES-tay
	Esta	ES-ta
That	Ese	ES-a
	Esa	ES-ah
These	Estos	ES-toes
	Estas	ES-tas
Those	Esos	ES-ohs
	Esas	ES-ahs
That one over there	Aquel	ah-**KEL**
	Aquellos	ah-**KAY**-yos
	Aquella	ah-**KAY**-ya
	Aquellas	ah-**KAY**-yas

Giving Colorful Commentary

Colors are important adjectives, and these words are very easy to use because you many already know many of them. Since these adjectives do not show possession or demonstrate one from another, they follow the same rules that the majority of adjectives do in Spanish. Position them after the noun they describe.

Colors must also "agree" with their nouns in two ways. First, by category: masculine or feminine. Next, your colors must agree in number: singular or plural. This is done by simply adding the letter "s" to the color so that it matches the plural ending (-s or –es) on the noun.

Los Colores

English	Español	Guide
Black	Negro	**NAY**-grow
Blue	Azul	ah-**SOOL**
Brown	Moreno	mo-**RAY**-no
Gold	Oro	**OH**-row
Gray	Gris	grease
Green	Verde	**VER**-day
Orange	Naranja	na-**RAHN**-ha
Pink	Rosa	**ROW**-sa
Purple	Morado	mo-**RAH**-do
Silver	Plata	**PLA**-ta
Red	Rojo	**ROW**-ho
White	Blanco	**BLAHN**-co
Yellow	Amarillo	ah-ma-**REE**-yo
Dark	Oscuro	ohs-**COO**-row
Light	Claro	**CLA**-row

What Is Your Complete Name?
¿CUÁL ES SU NOMBRE COMPLETO?

Hispanic Names Have Four Important Parts

First Name Primer Nombre	Middle Name Segundo Nombre	Father's Surname Apellido Paterno	Mother's Surname Apellido Materno
Carlos	Juan	Santana	Rodríguez
Ramón	Marco	Villarosa	Cruz

One of the most common errors in recording Hispanic names involves an incorrect understanding of their order. Many Hispanic "full" or "complete" names contain four parts: a first name, a middle or "second" name, and two family surnames.

The surname from an individual's paternal side is normally third in order. It is the correct choice for "last name" on forms instead of the name in the actual last position.

Look at the table containing names above. Santana, Villarosa, and Miranda are the correct choice for "last name." In many facilities both names are required. If that is the case in your institution, both names would be listed under last name. When alphabetizing, the third or paternal name would be used.

Do not insert an unnecessary hyphen between a man's *apellido paterno* and *apellido materno*. Hyphens are used in a married woman's name to show the linking of the two families. When addressing a Hispanic gentleman, it's correct to use either the *apellido paterno* alone or both family surnames.

Women:
A woman's name follows the same order and only changes upon marriage. When a single woman marries, she drops her *apellido materno* or "maiden" name. It is replaced by the *apellido paterno* of her husband.

Look closely at the following example:

Carmen Elena Miranda Rivera has married Carlos Juan Santana Rodríguez. She will now drop the use of her *apellido materno* which is "Rivera." She will add her husband's *apellido paterno* "Santana." Most women link their apellido paterno and their husbands with a hypen. Her name is now Carmen Miranda-Santana.

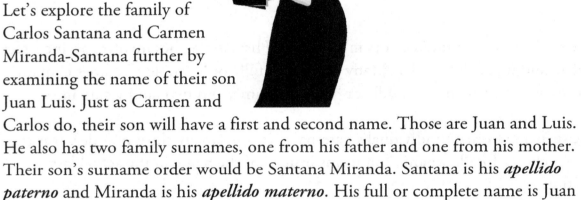

Children:
Let's explore the family of Carlos Santana and Carmen Miranda-Santana further by examining the name of their son Juan Luis. Just as Carmen and Carlos do, their son will have a first and second name. Those are Juan and Luis. He also has two family surnames, one from his father and one from his mother. Their son's surname order would be Santana Miranda. Santana is his *apellido paterno* and Miranda is his *apellido materno*. His full or complete name is Juan Luis Santana Miranda.

Full Name or Complete Name?

In any language there are usually at least three or four different ways to say just about anything you want to say. Both in Spanish and in English, there are at least three different ways to ask a person for their name. Here are the three most common ways to ask for this important bit of information:

1. ¿Cómo se llama?
2. ¿Cuál es su nombre?
3. ¿Cuál es su nombre completo?

If you choose option one, you are likely to receive only the individual's first name. Why? Because *cómo se llama* literally means "how do you call yourself. It does *not* mean what is your name.

Choice number two means what is your name, but, you are *still* not asking for the "whole enchilada"! Again, the person may only give you their name.

By using choice number three, you are asking for the person's full or complete name. In Spanish a person's entire name is always his or her "complete" name. It's never considered to be a "full" name. That's because for your name to technically be "full," it would also have to be the opposite of that or empty! Since your name doesn't hold water like a cup or food like your stomach does, your name can't possibly be full.

Your name is a piece of information, so it's considered to be either complete or incomplete. "*Completo*" is also a stronger match to the English word complete, making it much easier to use!

Spanish Nouns
Can words *really* have a gender?

¡Sí! Spanish belongs to the "romance" language family. It doesn't have anything to do with love, but it has a lot to do with the Romans. In ancient times, people had the same trouble learning languages that they do today — except that there were no cassette tapes, CDs, PDAs or very many foreign language teachers. In those days, there weren't many schools for that matter! Consequently, most folks were on their own when it came to learning another language.

To help the difficult process along, words were placed into categories based upon how they sounded. This process organized the material and made it easier to learn. Old world languages had categories that were often described as "masculine," "feminine," or even "neuter."

NOUN A person, place or thing

From these descriptions, people began talking about words in terms of their gender. Even though the word "gender" is misleading, the tendency to group words by sound helped people learn new languages more quickly.

Because Spanish evolved from Latin, it has maintained two category divisions for thousands of years. The categories are called masculine and feminine. Even though Spanish can and will evolve, the concept of categories in *español* is not likely to change.

Here are the most important points to remember about nouns and their categories:

1. Usually, the words are grouped by how they sound, not by what they mean. There will always be a few exceptions!

2. Languages are a lot like the people who use them: They don't always follow the rules!

3. If the Spanish noun is referring to a person, the letter will often indicate the sex of that individual. For example: a doctor, who is a man, is a "*doctor*," while a woman, who is a doctor, is a "*doctora*."

4. Words in the "masculine" category usually end with the letter "O".

5. Words in the "feminine" category usually end with the letter "A".

6. El, la, los and las are very important words. They all mean "the". They are the clues you need to tell you a word's category.

El (masculine category – singular)
Los (masculine category – plural)
La (feminine category – singular)
Las (feminine category – plural)

El niño, El muchacho
Los niños, Los muchachos
La niña, La muchacha
Las niñas, Las muchachas

TIPS & TIDBITS
Remember that learning the noun is the most important thing, not which category or gender it is! Words like "el" or "la" only mean "the." They don't give any clues to what you are trying to say. Learning the fine points of grammar can wait until you become a master of communications using Survival Spanish.

The Essentials of Spanish Verbs

There are basically three types of regular verbs in Spanish. The last two letters on the end of the verb determines how it is to be treated. Listed below are the three most common types of regular verb endings.

- ✓ **AR** – Hablar: To speak
- ✓ **ER** – Comprender: To understand
- ✓ **IR** – Escribir: To write

In Survival Spanish, we focus on speaking about ourselves and talking to another person. That's the most common type of "one-on-one" communication.

When you need to say I speak, I understand, or I live, change the last two letters of the verb to an "O".

- ✓ Hablo
- ✓ Comprendo
- ✓ Escribo

When asking a question, such as do you speak, do you understand, or do you live, change the ending to an "a" or an "e". *The change in letter indicates that you are speaking to someone else.*

- ✓ Habla
- ✓ Comprende
- ✓ Escribe

To make a sentence negative, simply put "no" in front of the verb.

- ✓ No hablo.
- ✓ No comprendo.
- ✓ No escribo.

VERB: Shows action or state of being

¡Acción!

There are so many English friendly *acción* words in the Spanish "AR" verb family. Many of them bear a strong resemblance to English verbs — most of them share a simple, regular nature. They are a very important asset in on-the-job communication. We picked a few of our favorites to get you started. Look closely at the list on the next page. On it you will recognize many comforting similarities between our languages that are practical too! Changing one letter will really expand your conversational skills.

In on-the-job conversations, people tend to use "I" and "you" to start many sentences. Of all the pronouns, these two are the most powerful and will work the best for you, so that's where we'll start.

Here's an important difference between our languages. In English, the use of pronouns is essential because most of our verbs tend to end the same way. For example, with I speak and you speak; the verb "speak" remains the same. In English, our pronouns make all the difference. Spanish is different in this aspect. Spanish-speaking people are listening for the letters on the end of the verb. That's what indicates who or what is being talked about in Spanish. Each ending is different. The end of the Spanish verb is much more important than the beginning. The ending of the verb tells the Spanish-speaking person who or what is being discussed. In most cases when people speak Spanish, you might not hear a pronoun. It's not necessary for precise meaning. That's a big reason why Spanish might sound a little fast to you: *Pronouns which are important in English are routinely eliminated in Spanish!*

Try this: Treat the verbs in the "AR" family as you would "to speak" or "hablar." End the verb with an "o" when you're talking about yourself; "hablo" or "I speak". Change the verb ending from an "o" to an "a" for "habla" or "you speak." Use this form when you're talking to someone else.

English	Español	Guide
I need	Necesito	nay-say-**SEE**-toe
You need	Necesita	nay-say-**SEE**-ta

The Sweet 16 Verbs

English	Español	Guide
1. To ask	Preguntar	prey-goon-**TAR**
2. To take	Tomar	toe-**MAR**
3. To call	Llamar	ya-**MAR**
4. To listen to	Escuchar	es-cooch-**ARE**
5. To cooperate	Cooperar	co-op-air-**RAR**
6. To forget	Olvidar	ohl-v-**DAR**
7. To fill	Llenar	yea-**NAR**
8. To need	Necesitar	nay-say-see-**TAR**
9. To observe	Observar	ob-ser-**VAR**
10. To pay	Pagar	pa-**GAR**
11. To prepare	Preparar	pray-pa-**RAR**
12. To return	Regresar	ray-grey-**SAR**
13. To verify	Verificar	ver-ree-fee-**CAR**
14. To use	Usar	oo-**SAR**
15. To look at	Mirar	me-**RAR**
16. To work	Trabajar	tra-baa-**HAR**

**Note: To make a sentence negative, say no in front of the verb.
   Example: I don't need. **No necesito.** You don't need **No necesita.**

Which verbs in the Sweet 16 do you use most often? List your top five:

1. _____

2. _____

3. _____

4. _____

5. _____

Now take your top five and change the AR ending to an "a" to indicate you are talking to someone else. Example: habla meaning you speak.

1. _____

2. _____

3. _____

4. _____

5. _____

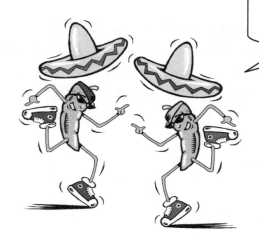

¡Necesito una breaka! ¿Y usted?

34

Irregular Verbs: The Big Five

Now that you have had the opportunity to learn about the tremendous number of verbs that follow regular patterns in Spanish, it's time to take a look at others that don't follow the rules. They are unpredictable, but they are very important. In fact, they reflect some of man's oldest concepts. That's why they tend to be irregular. These words were in use long before language rules and patterns were set. There are two verbs in Spanish that mean "to be." The others are: to have, to make and to go. Because they don't follow the rules, you will need to memorize them, but that should be easy because you will use and hear them often.

In English, the "to be" verb is I am, you are, he is, etc. The Spanish version is **ser** and **estar**. *Ser* is used to express permanent things like your nationality or profession. *Estar* is used when talking about location or conditions that change like a person's health.

Ser

Yo **soy**	Nosotros **somos**
Tú **eres**	
Él **es**	Ellos **son**
Ella **es**	Ellas **son**
Usted **es**	Ustedes **son**

Estar

Yo **estoy**	Nosotros **estamos**
Tú **estás**	
Él **está**	Ellos **están**
Ella **está**	Ellas **están**
Usted **está**	Ustedes **están**

The verb *"to have"* in Spanish, is *muy importante*. In English, we say that we are hot, cold, hungry, thirsty, right, wrong or sleepy, but in Spanish those are conditions that you have. Some of those expressions mean something totally different than you expected if you get the verbs confused, so be careful!

Tener

Yo **tengo**	Nosotros **tenemos**
Tú **tienes**	
Él **tiene**	Ellos **tienen**
Ella **tiene**	Ellas **tienen**
Usted **tiene**	Ustedes **tienen**

In Spanish, the verb that means *"to do"* also means *"to make."* It's not unusual for one verb to have multiple meanings. There are many expressions that require the use of this verb, but you will use it most when you talk about the weather. That's a safe subject and one that everyone the world over, discusses! **¿Qué tiempo hace?** What's the weather? **Hace frío.** (It's cold.) **Hace sol.** (It's sunny). **Hace calor.** (It's hot) **Hace viento** (It's windy.). Here are two exceptions: **Está lloviendo.** (It's raining.) and **Está nevando.** (It's snowing.)

Hacer

Yo **hago**	Nosotros **hacemos**
Tú **haces**	
Él **hace**	Ellos **hacen**
Ella **hace**	Ellas **hacen**
Usted **hace**	Ustedes **hacen.**

The last of the big five is perhaps the easiest to use. It's the verb that means, *"to go"*. In Spanish, that's **ir**. It's pronounced like the English word ear. Both in English and in Spanish, we use parts of it to make the future tense, in other words, to talk about things that we are going to do. Look at the parts of *ir*. Then look back at the parts of the verb *ser*. Do you notice any similarities?

Ir

Yo **voy**	Nosotros **vamos**
Tú **vas**	
Él **va**	Ellos **van**
Ella **va**	Ellas **van**
Usted **va**	Ustedes **van**

When you want to say something that you are going to do, start with I'm going or *voy*. Next, insert the word *"a"* and the basic verb that states what it is that you're going to do. Try it! It's easy. Here are some examples.

Voy a llamar a su doctor.	I am going to call your doctor.
Voy a explicar los efectos adversos.	I am going to explain the side effects.
Mario va a comprar la medicina.	Mario is going to buy the medicine.

Note: The whole concept of irregular verbs can be quite daunting. Don't let it defeat you! We have many irregular verbs in English. Every language has them. The only way to master them is to use them. Make them your own! Try writing different parts of a verb on your desk calendar. That way, it will be there in front of you every time you look down. When you see it, say it to yourself. Then, you'll have it conquered in no time.

Are you hungry? — ¿Tiene hambre?

Using the right verb at the right time is very important. The following common expressions in Spanish require the use of *tener*. These are phrases you must learn, even though the translation will feel strange to you. *Remember our English idioms often sound very strange to others.* As a rule, *tener* is used to describe physical conditions. In English we use the verb *to be.*

TENER: To have   **TENGO: I have**   **TIENE: You have**

English	Español	Guide
Hot	Calor	ca-**LORE**
Hungry	Hambre	**AM**-bray
Cold	Frío.	**FREE**-oh
Ashamed	Vergüenza	ver-goo-**N**-sa
In pain.	Dolor	doe-**LORE**
Afraid of	Miedo de	me-**A**-doe day
Right	Razón	rah-**SEWN**
Thirsty	Sed	said
Sleepy	Sueño	soo-**WAYNE**-nyo
xx years old	*xx* años	**AHN**-yos

What's the Weather? — ¿Qué tiempo hace?

No matter what the culture is a general topic for discussion is always the weather. Discussing the weather in Spanish requires a different verb from the one used in English. If you say to your host, "*Está frío*," he or she would think that you were talking about something you had touched. In Spanish, use the verb **hacer** which means to do or to make to describe the weather. It's one of the big five irregulars.

English	Español	Guide
Rain	Lluvia	U-v-ah
To be cold	Hace frío	**AH**-say **FREE**-oh
To be cool	Hace fresco	**AH**-say **FRES**-co
To be hot	Hace calor	**AH**-say ca-**LORE**
To be nice weather	Hace buen tiempo	**AH**-say boo-**WAYNE** t-**M**-po
To be sunny	Hace sol	**AH**-say sol
To be windy	Hace viento	**AH**-say v-**N**-toe
To rain.	Llover	**YO**-ver
What's the weather?	¿Qué tiempo hace?	kay t-**M**-poe **AH**-say

TIPS & TIDBITS

In North America we use the Fahrenheit scale for measuring the temperature. Latin American countries use the Celsius scale. What's the difference? Here's a simple example: 0 degrees Celsius is 32 degrees Fahrenheit.

Special Uses of Ser and Estar

The verbs *ser* and *estar* both mean the same thing in English: *to be,* but *how can two verbs mean the same thing?* It's because *ser* and *estar* are used in very different ways. Spanish sees these two verbs differently and uses them in very precise ways. Listed below are some simple guidelines on their usage:

COMMON USES OF SER

A. To express an permanent quality or characteristic

La puerta es de madera.	The door is made of wood.
El hospital es enorme.	The hospital is enormous.
Los farmacéuticos son importantes.	Pharmacists are important.

B. To describe or identify

Mi amigo es un doctor.	My friend is a doctor.
El paciente es alto.	The patient is tall.

C. To indicate nationality

El doctor es mexicano.	The doctor is Mexican.
La historia es de Argentina.	The story is from Argentina.

D. To express ownership

Este es mi receta médica	This is my prescription.
Este es mi libro.	This is my book.

E. To express time and dates

¿Qué hora es?	What time is it?
Hoy es el nueve de junio.	Today is the 9th of June.

F.   With impersonal expressions.

Es importante estudiar.   It's important to study.

Es necesario leer las instrucciones.   It's necessary read the instructions.

COMMON USES OF ESTAR

A.   To express location

Estoy en la oficina.   I am in the office.

Charlotte está en Carolina del Norte. Charlotte is in North Carolina.

El baño está en el segundo piso.   The bathroom is on the 2nd floor.

B.   To indicate someone's health

Mi esposa está enferma.   My wife is sick.

¿Cómo está usted?   How are you?

C.   *Estar* is also used as a helping verb

Estoy hablando.   I am speaking.

Carmen está trabajando.   Carmen is working.

Julio está regresando mañana.   Julio is returning tomorrow.

TIPS & TIDBITS

Notice from the examples that *ser* is used more frequently than *estar*. Even though the usage of *ser* and *estar* seems complicated in the beginning, both verbs are used so frequently in conversation that you will become comfortable using them quickly.

The Numbers — Los Números

Number	Español	Guide
0	Cero	**SAY**-row
1	Uno	**OO**-no
2	Dos	dose
3	Tres	trays
4	Cuatro	coo-**AH**-trow
5	Cinco	**SINK**-oh
6	Seis	**SAY**-ees
7	Siete	see-**A**-tay
8	Ocho	**OH**-cho
9	Nueve	new-**A**-vay
10	Diez	d-**ACE**
11	Once	**ON**-say
12	Doce	**DOSE**-a
13	Trece	**TRAY**-say
14	Catorce	ca-**TOR**-say
15	Quince	**KEEN**-say
16	Diez y seis	d-**ACE** e **SAY**-ees
17	Diez y siete	d-**ACE** e see-**ATE**-tay
18	Diez y ocho	d-**ACE** e **OH**-cho
19	Diez y nueve	d-**ACE** e new-**A**-vay
20	Veinte	**VAIN**-tay
21	Veinte y uno	**VAIN**-tay e **OO**-no
22	Veinte y dos	**VAIN**-tay e dose

Number	Español	Guide
23	Veinte y tres	**VAIN**-tay e trays
24	Veinte y cuatro	**VAIN**-tay e coo-**AH**-trow
25	Veinte y cinco	**VAIN**-tay e **SINK**-oh
26	Veinte y seis	**VAIN**-tay e **SAY**-ees
27	Veinte y siete	**VAIN**-tay e see-**A**-tay
28	Veinte y ocho	**VAIN**-tay e **OH**-cho -
29	Veinte y nueve	**VAIN**-tay e new-**A**-vay
30	Treinta	**TRAIN**-ta
40	Cuarenta	kwah-**RAIN**-ta
50	Cincuenta	seen-**KWAIN**-ta
60	Sesenta	say-**SAIN**-ta
70	Setenta	say-**TAIN**-ta
80	Ochenta	oh-**CHAIN**-ta
90	Noventa	no-**VAIN**-ta
100	Cien	see-**IN**
200	Doscientos	dose-see-**N**-toes
300	Trescientos	tray-see-**N**-toes
400	Cuatrocientos	coo-**AH**-troh-see-**N**-toes
500	Quinientos	keen-e-**N**-toes
600	Seiscientos	**SAY**-ees-see-**N**-toes
700	Setecientos	**SAY**-tay-see-**N**-toes
800	Ochocientos	**OH**-choh- see-**N**-toes
900	Novecientos	**NO**-vay-see-**N**-toes
1,000	Mil	meal

Days of the Week and Months of the Year
Los Días de la Semana

English	Español	Guide
Monday	lunes	LOON-ace
Tuesday	martes	MAR-tays
Wednesday	miércoles	me-AIR-co-lace
Thursday	jueves	who-WAVE-ace
Friday	viernes	v-AIR-nace
Saturday	sábado	SAH-ba-doe
Sunday	domingo	doe-MING-go

**When expressing a date in Spanish, give the number of the day first.
Follow the day with the month. Use this format:
El (date) de (month).**

The Months of the Year
Los Meses del Año

English	Español	Guide
January	enero	n-NAY-row
February	febrero	fay-BRAY-row
March	marzo	MAR-so
April	abril	ah-BRILL
May	mayo	MY-oh
June	junio	WHO-knee-oh
July	julio	WHO-lee-oh
August	agosto	ah-GOSE-toe
September	septiembre	sep-tee-EM-bray
October	octubre	oc-TOO-bray
November	noviembre	no-v-EM-bray
December	diciembre	d-see-EM-bray

**Your appointment is (day of the week) el (number) de (month).
Su cita es lunes, el 11 de octubre.**

Practicing Numbers & Dates

Practice these important items by using numbers, days of the week, and months of the year:

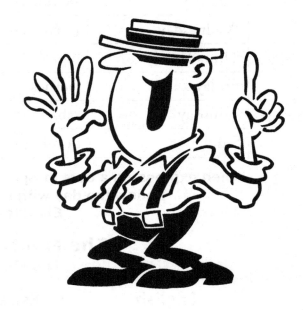

- ✓ Your social security number

- ✓ Your driver's license number

- ✓ The numbers in your address

- ✓ Your zip code

- ✓ Your phone number

- ✓ Your birth date

- ✓ Your children's birth dates

- ✓ The dates of holidays

- ✓ License tags of the cars in front of you, when you are stopped in traffic.

Combine the Spanish alphabet with this exercise.

- ✓ Phone numbers you see on billboards

- ✓ Numbers found on street signs

- ✓ Phone numbers when you dial them at work or at home

- ✓ The appointments on your personal calendar

- ✓ Your wedding anniversary

- ✓ The dates of all your Spanish classes or practice sessions

What Time Is It? — ¿Qué Hora Es?

The concept of time is something that varies from culture to culture. Many countries put less emphasis on being on time for certain things than Americans do. In Latino culture one lives for the present. It can be especially true in one's personal life; however, on the job everyone knows the value of *puntualidad*. *¡Es muy importante!*

Learning to tell time is another good way to put your numbers in Spanish to good use *¿Qué hora es?* means *what time is it?*

It's one o'clock.	Es la una.
It's two o'clock.	Son las dos.
It's 3:30.	Son las tres y media.
It's 5:45.	Son las seis menos quince.

Use the phrases *de la mañana* to indicate morning and *de la tarde* to indicate afternoon. Also midnight is *medianoche*. Noon is *mediodía*.

To find out at what time something takes place ask: *¿A qué hora…?*

¿A qué hora es la reunión?	What time is the meeting?
¿A qué hora termina?	What time do you finish?

Spanish speakers sometimes use the 24-hour clock for departures and arrivals of trains and flights, etc.

12:05	las doce cero cinco
17.52	las diez y siete cincuenta y dos
23.10	las veinte y tres diez
07.15	las siete quince

Para Practicar

1. Using the word for meeting "*la reunion*," say that your meeting takes place on the hour throughout your workday. *La reunión es a las ocho.*

Scheduling an Appointment

When you need to schedule an appointment, this form will come in very handy for you. In *español* an appointment is called a *cita* (SEE-ta). List the name of the individual that the appointment is with first. Then circle the day of the week and add the number for the day. Finally, circle the month and add the time. The phrase at the bottom of this form simply asks the individual to arrive ten minutes early for the appointment.

Usted tiene una cita importante con _____.

La cita es   lunes   el _____ de   enero   a las _____.

               martes   febrero

               miércoles   marzo

               jueves   abril

               viernes   mayo

                                                 junio

                                                 julio

                                                 agosto

                                                 septiembre

                                                 octubre

                                                 noviembre

                                                 diciembre

**Favor de llegar 10 minutos antes del tiempo de su cita. ¡Gracias!*

Please arrive 10 minutes before the time of your appointment. Thank you.

The Questions Everyone Should Know

English	Español	Guide
Who?	¿Quién?	key-**N**
What?	¿Qué?	kay
Which?	¿Cuál?	coo-**ALL**
When?	¿Cuándo?	**KWAN**-doe
Where?	¿Dónde?	**DON**-day
Why?	¿Por qué?	pour **KAY**
How?	¿Cómo?	**CO**-mo
What's happening?	¿Qué pasa?	kay **PA**-sa
How much?	¿Cuánto?	**KWAN**-toe
How many?	¿Cuántos?	**KWAN**-toes

When you ask a question in Spanish, it will take on the same form as a question does in English. Start with the question word that asks the information you need. Follow the question word with a verb, and give your voice an upward inflection.

In Spanish you can also make a question by ending your sentence with ¿no? Here's an example: *Cancún está en México, ¿no?* When you end a sentence with "no" like this, it takes on the meaning of "isn't it."

The Most Common Questions

How are you?   ¿Cómo está?
How much does it cost?   ¿Cuánto cuesta?
Where are you from?   ¿De dónde es?

> To make the Spanish upside down question mark or the upside down exclamation mark refer, to the chapter called "Typing in Spanish on Your Computer."

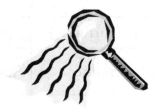

Getting the Información

Listed below are common phrases which are used to fill out almost any questionnaire. It seems like most forms ask for the same information in almost the same order. By learning a few simple phrases, you can use this format to your advantage.

There are so many times when we need to ask for very basic information. Most of these questions begin with the words *what is your.* When you are asking this type of question, remember that it's not always necessary to make a complete sentence to have good communication. The information you are asking for is much more important than the phrase "what is your"? As long as you remember to make what you say *sound* like a question by giving your voice an *upward* inflection, people will interpret what you've said *as* a question.

Use the form on the following page. It asks for very basic information. To help you practice, work with a partner. Make up new information about yourself and complete the form. At each practice session one of you will ask the questions and the other will give the answers to fill in the information requested. This is a great practice exercise, because when you think about it, most of the time the questions you ask will be the same, but the answers you get will always be different!

What's your. . .   ¿Cuál es su. . .
coo-ALL es sue

English	Español	Guide
Full name	Nombre completo	NOM-bray com-PLAY-toe
First name	Primer nombre	pre-MARE NOM-bray
Middle name	Segundo nombre	say-GOON-doe NOM-bray
Last name (surname)	Apellido	ah-pay-YE-doe
Paternal surname	Apellido paterno	ah-pay-YE-doe pa-TER-no

English	Español	Guide
Maternal surname	Apellido materno	ah-pay-YE-doe ma-TER-no
Address	Dirección	d-wreck-see-ON
Apartment number	Número de apartamento	NEW-may-row day ah-par-ta-MEN-toe
Age	Edad	a-DAD
Date of birth	Fecha de nacimiento	FAY-cha day na-see-me-N-toe
Nationality	Nacionalidad	na-see-on-nal-e-DAD
Place of birth	Lugar de nacimiento	loo-GAR day na-see-me-N-toe
Place of employment	Lugar de empleo	loo-GAR day m-PLAY-oh
Occupation	Ocupación	oh-coo-pa-see-ON
Home telephone number	Número de teléfono de su casa	NEW-may-row day tay-LAY-fo-no day sue CA-sa
Work telephone number	Número de teléfono de su empleo	NEW-may-row day tay-LAY-fo-no day sue m-PLAY-oh
Marital status	Estado civil	es-TA-doe see-VEAL
Married	Casado (a)	ca-SA-doe
Single	Soltero (a)	soul-TAY-row
Divorced	Divorciado (a)	d-vor-see-AH-doe
Widow	Viudo (a)	v-OO-doe
Separated	Separado (a)	sep-pa-RAH-doe
Driver's license number	Número de licencia	NEW-may-row day lee-SEN-see-ah
Social security number	Número de seguro social	NEW-may-row day say-GOO-row sew-see-AL

Información Básica
Imprima por favor

Fecha: _____
                               Mes   Día   Año

Sr.
Sra.
Srta. _____
       Primer Nombre   *Segundo Nombre*   *Apellido Paterno*   *Apellido Materno (Esposo)*

Dirección: _____
                                        Calle

_____
Ciudad   *Estado*   *Zona postal*

Teléfono: Casa _____   **Empleo** _____

            Cel _____   **Fax** _____

Correo electrónico _____

Número de seguro social: _____-_____-_____

Fecha de nacimiento _____
                             Mes   Día   Año

Número de la licencia: _____

Ocupación: _____

Lugar de empleo _____

Estado civil: Casado (a)
                  Soltero (a)
                  Divorciado (a)
                  Separado (a)
                  Viudo (a)

Nombre de esposo: _____
          Primer Nombre   *Segundo Nombre* *Apellido Paterno*   *Apellido Materno*
Nombre de esposa: _____
        Primer Nombre   *Segundo Nombre* *Apellido Paterno*   *Apellido Materno/Esposo*

En caso de emergencia: _____ **Teléfono:** _____

Firma: _____   **Fecha:** _____

See page 108 for an English translation of the basic information form.

50

The Family — La Familia

Putting our families first is something all Americans have in common. It is especially true for Latinos. For them, family values are extremely important. No sacrifice is too great if it helps the family. Children are considered to be precious gifts. Wives, mothers and grandmothers are highly respected. Remember, that the maternal side of the family is so important that traditionally Hispanics carry their mother's surname or *materno apellido* as a part of their complete name. If you have forgotten the four important parts of a Latino's name, please review the chapter called *"Cuál es su nombre completo."*

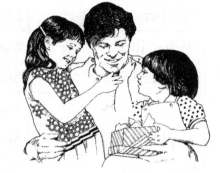

You are certainly going to hear about members of the family from your Hispanic customers. It's something all of us like to talk about!

English	Español	Guide
Aunt	Tía	T-ah
Uncle	Tío	T-oh
Brother	Hermano	air-**MAN**-oh
Sister	Hermana	air-**MAN**-ah
Brother-in-law	Cuñado	coon-**YA**-doe
Sister-in-law	Cuñada	coon-**YA**-da
Child	Niño *(m)* Niña *(f)*	**KNEE**-nyo **KNEE**-nya
Cousin	Primo *(m)* Prima *(f)*	**PRE**-mo **PRE**-ma
Daughter	Hija	E-ha
Son	Hijo	E-ho

English	Español	Guide
Daughter-in-law	Nuera	new-**AIR**-rah
Son-in-law	Yerno	**YAIR**-no
Father	Padre	**PA**-dray
Mother	Madre	**MA**-dray
Father-in-law	Suegro	soo-**A**-grow
Mother-in-law	Suegra	soo-**A**-gra
Niece	Sobrina	so-**BREE**-na
Nephew	Sobrino	so-**BREE**-no
Step father	Padrastro	pa-**DRAS**-tro
Step mother	Madrastra	ma-**DRAS**-tra
Step son	Hijastro	e-**HAS**-tro
Step daughter	Hijastra	e-**HAS**-tra
Granddaughter	Nieta	knee-**A**-ta
Grandson	Nieto	knee-**A**-toe
Grandfather	Abuelo	ah-boo-**A**-low
Grandmother	Abuela	ah-boo-**A**-la
Husband	Esposo	es-**POE**-so
Wife	Esposa	es-**POE**-sa

TIPS & TIDBITS

The Hispanic family is a very close-kit group. The term *familia* goes beyond the nuclear family and includes not only parents and children but the entire extended family. In traditional Hispanic families, the father is the "head of the household" and the mother is responsible for the home. Individual family members have a responsibility to aid others in the family when they experience financial problems — or a health crisis. One can always depend on one's *familia*.

People in the Hospital
Personas en el hospital

A hospital pharmacists' role in the healthcare setting is different from that of a retail pharmacist. If you work in a hospital, at some point, you will run into a visitor or a patient who will ask you about members of the hospital staff. Here are some important members of the medical team. This is a much easier list since so many of the words are almost the same as they are in English.

Work steadily and slowly on your Spanish. The key to fluency is practice! Don't let it overwhelm you! Remember the story about the race between the tortoise and the hare? The tortoise kept a slow steady pace and finished the race, while the hare burned himself out by not pacing himself. Try for one word each day. Keep sticky notes in your car, along with a pen. Put one new word or phrase on the steering wheel of your car first thing every morning. Every time you stop, take a look at the word of the day. Try to use it in a conversation during the day. By keeping a slow steady pace like this, you will be comfortable in a few short months.

English	Español	Guide
Assistant	Ayudante	ay-oo-**DAN**-tay
Boss	Jefe	**HEF**-a
	Jefa	**HEF**-ah
Child	Niño	**NEEN**-yo
	Niña	**NEEN**-ya
Doctor	Doctor	doc-**TOR**
	Doctora	doc-**TOR**-rah

English	Español	Guide
Housekeeper	Doméstico *(a)*	doe-**MAYS**-tee-co
In-patient	Paciente interno	pa-see-**N**-tay n-**TER**-no
Janitor	Portero *(a)*	pour-**TAY**-row
Nurse	Enfermera *(o)*	n-fair-**MARE**-rah
Out-patient	Paciente externo	pa-see-**N**-tay x-**TER**-no
Paramedic	Paramédico	para-**MAY**-d-co
Patient	Paciente	pa-see-**N**-tay
Pharmacist	Farmacéutico *(a)*	far-ma-**SAY**-oo-t-co
Police	Policía	poe-lee-**SEE**-ah
Receptionist	Recepcionista	ray-cept-see-on-**KNEES**-ta
Secretary	Secretaria	sec-ree-**TAR**-ree-ah
Security guard	Guardia de seguridad	goo-**ARE**-dee-ah day say-goo-ree-**DAD**
Supervisor	Supervisor	soo-pear-**V**-soar
	Supervisora	soo-pear-v-**SOAR**-ah
Therapist	Terapeuta	terra-pay-**OO**-ta
Visitor	Visitante	v-see-**TAN**-tay

TIPS & TIDBITS

With Hispanics verbal and nonverbal communication is characterized by *respeto* (respect). There is an element of formality in their interactions especially when older persons are involved. Over-familiarity such as the touch of a stranger or the casual use of one's first name is not appreciated early in the relationship. A brisk "business-like" approach could inhibit you from finding out a patient's complaint — and you may find that this patient is less likely to return for treatment.

Places in the Hospital — Lugares en el Hospital

If you are a hospital pharmacist, you will need to know how to give directions to places in the hospital. Here is a list of departments or *departamentos* in the hospital. Notice that many of the hospital's departments are similar to English, but remember to say the full name of the department rather than using abbreviations like ER and ICU. People that are new to speaking English won't know what these letters stand for!

English	Español	Guide
Basement	Sótano	**SO**-tan-oh
Cafeteria	Cafetería	ca-fay-ter-**REE**-ah
Department	Departamento	day-par-ta-**MEN**-toe
Elevator	Ascensor	ah-sen-**SOAR**
Emergency room	Sala de emergencia	**SAL**-la day a-mare-**HEN**-see ah
Entrance	Entrada	in-**TRA**-dah
Exit	Salida	sal-**LEE**-da
Gift shop	Tienda de regalos	t-**N**-da day ray-**GAL**-os
Hall	Corredor	core-ray-**DOOR**
Intensive care	Cuidados intensivos	kwe-**DA**-does n-ten-**SEE**-vows
Laboratory	Laboratorio	lab-oh-rah-**TOR**-e-oh
Lobby	Salón	sal-**ON**
Maternity	Maternidad	ma-ter-knee-**DAD**
Operating room	Sala de operacione	**SAL**-la day oh-pear-rah-see-**ON**
Parking lot	Estacionamiento	es-ta-see-on-ah-me-**N**-toe

English	Español	Guide
Pediatrics	Pediátrico	pay-d-**AH**-tree-co
Physical therapy	Terapia física	ter-**RAH**-p-ah **FEE**-see-ka
Radiology	Radiología	rah-d-oh-low-**HE**-ah
Recovery room	Sala de recuperación	**SAL**-la day ray-coo-pear-ra-see-**ON**
Respiratory therapy	Terapia respiratoria	ter-**RAH**-p-ah res-pier-ah-**TOR**-e-ah
Rest room	Sanitario Baño	san-knee-**TAR**-ree-o **BAN**-yo
Stairs	Escaleras	es-ka-**LAIR**-as
Telephone	Teléfono	tay-**LAY**-fono
Waiting room	Sala de espera	**SAL**-la day es-**PEAR**-ah
Water fountain	Fuente de agua	foo-**N**-tay day **AH**-gua
X-ray	Rayos equis	rah-yos **A**-kees

Giving Directions

The ability to give directions in *español* is one of the most practical skills you can have. As you direct clients from one agency to another, these words will really be a *grande* plus to your conversational ability, you will definitely use these words over and over again. Slowly, you can start to learn this important vocabulary by knowing simple things, such as the four directions: north, south, east and west. Then, add turns like right and left. Before you know it, you'll be able to give directions to places around town and in your office. This practical vocabulary is easy to practice because you can work on it anywhere you go!

English	Español	Guide
Where is…?	¿Dónde está…?	**DON**-day es-**TA**
Above	Encima	n-**SEE**-ma
Aisle	Pasillo	pa-**SEE**-yo
Avenue	Avenida	ah-ven-**KNEE**-da
Behind	Detrás	day-**TRAHS**
Beside	Al lado de	al **LA**-doe day
Down	Abajo	ah-**BAA**-ho
East	Este	**ES**-tay
Far	Lejos	**LAY**-hos
Here	Aquí	ah-**KEY**
In front of	En frente de	n **FREN**-tay day
Inside	Adentro	ah-**DEN**-tro
Near	Cerca de	**CER**-ca day
North	Norte	**NOR**-tay
Outside	Afuera	ah-foo-**AIR**-ah
Over there	Allá	ah-**YA**
South	Sur	**SUE**-er
Straight ahead	Adelante	ah-day-**LAN**-tay
Street	Calle	ca-**YEA**
There	Allí	ah-**YE**
To the left	A la izquierda	ah la ees-key-**AIR**-dah
To the right	A la derecha	ah la day-**RAY**-cha
Turn	Doble	**DOE**-blay
Up	Arriba	ah-**REE**-ba
West	Oeste	oh-**ES**-tay

Neither the names of businesses nor the names of streets are translated into Spanish. The proper name of your agency is its brand or trade-mark and should not be translated. Consequently, the name of a street is its proper or given name and should not be translated either.

In most Latin American cities, numbers and the words street and avenue are commonly used in addresses as they are in most metropolitan areas of the US. It's not uncommon to find 5th Avenue or 52nd Street. But, our neighborhood streets…well, that's another story entirely! Street names like Taniger Lane, Red Fox Run, or Wood Stork Cove are impossible to translate from one language to another. You should be aware, however, that sometimes a Spanish-speaking person will give you the number of their street address *en español*. Simple numbers are one of the most important sets of vocabulary you can have!

Instructions - Instrucciones

Here are some common instructions for the workplace. Whether you are behind the counter, speaking with customers or working with store employees these phrases will help you communicate in a variety of situations. Don't forget to add *gracias* or *por favor* at the beginning or at the end of the phrase.

English	Español	Guide
Come here	Venga aquí	**VEN**-ga ah-**KEY**
Let's go	Vámonos	**VA**-mo-nos
Go with him	Vaya con él	**VA**-ya con L
Wait	Espere	ace-**PEAR**-ray
Stop	Pare	**PAR**-ray
Help me	Ayúdeme	ay-**U**-day-may
Help him	Ayúdelo	ay-**U**-day-low

English	Español	Guide
Like this	Así	ah-**SEE**
Not like this	Así no	ah-**SEE** no
Show me	Muéstreme	moo-**ACE**-tray-may
Good	Bien	b**N**
Point to it	Indícalo.	n-**DEE**-ka-low
Move that here	Mueve eso aquí	moo-wavy **ES**-so ah-**KEY**
Bring me that	Tráigame eso.	try-**GA**-may **ES**-toe
Give it to me	Démelo.	**DAY**-may-low
To the right	A la derecha	a la day-**RAY**-cha
To the left	A la izquierda.	a la ees-kay-**AIR**-da
Remove these	Quite estos	**KEY**-tay **ES**-toes
Pick up all these	Recoja todo esto	ray-**CO**-ha **TOE**-dos **ES**-toes
Put it there	Póngalo allí	**PON**-ga-low ah-**YE**
Around	Alrededor	al-ray-day-**DOOR**
Inside	Dentro	**DEN**-tro
Under	Debajo	day-**BA**-ho
Carry this.	Lleve esto	**YEA**-vay **ACE**-toe
Open/close	Abre, cierra	**AH**-bray. **SER**-ray
Do it now.	Hágalo ahora.	**AH**-ga-low ah-**ORA**
Do it later.	Hágalo más tarde	**AH**-ga-low mas **TAR**-day
Here, there	Aquí, allí	ah-**KEY**, ah-**YE**
A little, a lot	Un poco, mucho	un **PO**-ko, **MOO**-cho

In English it's common to say, "Do you understand my directions? In Spanish, remember to always use the word **instructions** instead of **directions.** This could be confusing to some Latinos because the word *dirección* in español can mean *address!* It's a good idea to ask this simple question: *¿Comprende mis instrucciones?* Also, don't forget to add *por favor* or please to your *instrucciones!*

On the Telephone

Talking on the telephone with Spanish-speaking patients, customers or family members is one of the most challenging skills to develop. There's no body language or facial expression from the person on the other end of the line to help you. The best way to start this process is to stay as organized as possible. Think carefully about the kind of calls you make to your English speaking customers. What are the phrases you say most often to them and the typical responses you receive? These are probably going to be many of the same questions your Spanish-speaking patients ask too, so learn those key phrases first.

Remember it's better to use some of the phrases from page 15 to help you if you get in a jam. There's nothing wrong with saying, *"Repeta, por favor. Habla más despacio."* Make a script to help you get started building your telephone skills. A script or other notes will help you build your confidence— and that's *muy importante!*.

English	Español	Guide
800 number	Número de ochocientos	NEW-may-row day OH-cho-see-N-toes
Answering machine	Contestador telefónico	con-tes-TA-door tay-lay-FO-knee-co

English	Español	Guide
Area code	Código de área	**CO**-d-go day **AH**-ray-ah
Ask for this number.	Pida este número.	p-da **ES**-tay **NEW**-may-row
Cellular phone	Teléfono celular

El cel | tay-lay-**FO**-no say-**YOU**-lar

el cell |
Collect call	Llamada a cobro revertido	ya-**MA**-da ah **CO**-bro ray-ver-**T**-doe
Conference call	Llamada de conferencia	ya-**MA**-da de con-fer-**WRENN**-see-ah
Could you call later?	¿Puede llamar más tarde?	poo-**A**-day ya-**MAR** mas **TAR**-day
Dial this number.	Marque este número.	**MAR**-que **ES**-tay **NEW**-may-row
Extension	Extensión	x-ten-see-**ON**
Fax	Facsímile	fax-**SEE**-meal
Hang up the telephone.	Cuelgue el teléfono.	coo-**L**-gay el tay-**LAY**-foe-no
He/She isn't here.	No está aquí.	no es-**TA** ah-**KEY**
He/she will call back later.	Llamará más tarde.	ya-**MAR**-rah **MAS** tar-**DAY**
Headset	Auriculares con micrófono	ow-ree-coo-**LAR**-es con me-**CROW**-foe-no
Hold a moment,	Espere un momento, por favor.	es-**PEAR**-ray oon mo-**MEN**-toe pour fa-**VOR**
I have the wrong number.	Tengo el número equivocado.	**TANG**-go el **NEW**-may-row a-key-vo-**CA**-doe

English	Español	Guide
I'd like to leave a message.	Me gustaría dejar un mensaje.	may goo-star-**REE**-ah day-**HAR** oon men-**SA**-je
I'll transfer you to _____	Le voy a transferir a _____	lay voy a trans-fair-**REAR** ah
I'm calling about_____.	Estoy llamando acerca de _____.	es-**TOY** ya-**MAHN**-doe ah-**SER**-ca day
Is this the correct number?	¿Es el número correcto?	es el **NEW**-may-row co-**WRECK**-toe
It's very important.	Es muy importante.	es mooy m-pour-**TAHN**-tay
Local call	Llamada local	ya-**MA**-da low-**CAL**
Long distance	Larga distancia	**LAR**-ga dees-**TAN**-see-ah
May I speak to _____?	¿Puedo hablar con _____?	poo-**A**-doe ah-**BLAR** con _____
Press this number.	Oprima este número.	oh-**PRE**-ma **ES**-tay **NEW**-may-row
Repeat that please.	Repítelo, por favor	ray-**P**-tay-low pour fa-**VOR**
Switchboard	Conmutador	con-moo-ta-**DOOR**
Telephone number	Número de teléfono	**NEW**-may-row day tay-**LAY**-foe-no
The connection is bad.	La conexión está mala.	la co-nex-see-**ON** es-**TA MA**-la
The line is busy.	La línea está ocupada.	la **LEE**-nay-ah es-**TA** oh-coo-**PA**-da
The number is disconnected.	El número está desconectado.	el **NEW**-may-row es-**TA** des-co-neck-**TA**-da
There is a phone call for _____	Hay una llamada para _____.	eye **OO**-na ya-**MA**-da **PA**-ra _____.

English	Español	Guide
Two-way radio	Radioteléfono portátil	ra-d-oh-tay-**LAY**-foe-no pour-**TA**-teel
Wait for the tone.	Espere por el tono.	es-**PEAR**-ray pour el **TOE**-no
Would you like to leave a message?	¿Le gustaría dejar un mensaje?	lay goo-star-**REE**-ah day-**HAR** oon men-**SA**-he
You have the wrong number.	Tiene el número equivocado.	t-**N**-a l **NEW**-may-row a-key-vo-**CA**-doe
Your name, please	Su nombre, por favor	sue **NOM**-brey pour fa-**VOR**
Your number, please	Su número, por favor	sue **NEW**-may-row pour fa-**VOR**

TIPS & TIDBITS

Speaking Spanish to a customer on the telephone is a skill that you can accomplish through careful planning and scripting. Before you pick up the telephone to dial, think carefully about what you want to say. This technique will keep you from being nervous and will make you more successful from your first attempt. Before you begin to dial, look up all the vocabulary words and phrases you will need. If you are leaving a message for a Spanish-speaking customer, make sure to say your name and the telephone number where you can be reached slowly and distinctly

Please Call a Doctor!   ¡Favor de llamar un doctor!

In situations where you are called upon to evaluate a patient's illness or injury, quick reactions and good communication are essential to handling the crisis. Your knowledge of these basic parts of human anatomy will give you and your patient confidence. Knowing them will also help you build trust with your patient and family members. Listed below are laymen's terms for the parts of the body. Because you will be dealing with Hispanics from all parts of the Spanish-speaking world, this list will help you communicate quickly with all of them. Learning these parts of the body will help you in emergency situations — and could help you save a life!

English	Español	Guide
Ankle	Tobillo	toe-**B**-yo
Arm	Brazo	**BRA**-so
Back	Espalda	es-**PALL**-doe
Body	Cuerpo	coo-**AIR**-poe
Brain	Cerebro	say-**RAY**-bro
Calf (of the leg)	Pantorilla	pan-tor-**REE**-ya
Cheek	Mejilla	may-**HE**-ya
Chest	Pecho	**PAY**-cho
Chin	Barbilla	bar-**B**-ya
Ear	Oreja	oh-**RAY**-ha
Eye	Ojo	**OH**-ho
Face	Cara	**CA**-ra
Finger	Dedo	**DAY**-do
Foot	Pie	**P**-ay
Forehead	Frente	**FREN**-tay
Hand	Mano	**MA**-no
Head	Cabeza	ca-**BAY**-sa
Heart	Corazón	core-ra-**SEWN**
Knee	Rodilla	row-**D**-ya
Ligament	Ligamento	lee-ga-**MEN**-toe
Leg	Pierna	p-**YAIR**-na

English	Español	Guide
Mouth	Boca	**BOW**-ca
Nail	Uña	**OON**-ya
Neck	Cuello	coo-**A**-yo
Nose	Nariz	na-**REECE**
Skin	Piel	p-**L**
Shin	Espinilla	es-pee-**KNEE**-ya
Shoulder	Hombro	**ON**-bro
Spine	Espina	ace-**P**-na
Stomach	Estómago	ace-**TOE**-ma-go
Tendon	Tendón	ten-**DON**
Throat	Garganta	gar-**GAN**-ta
Toe	Dedo del pie	**DAY**-doe del **P**-a
Tooth	Diente	d-**N**-tay
Wrist	Muñeca	moon-**YEA**-ca

The Eyes — Los Ojos

English	Español	Guide
Eye	ojo	**OH**-ho
Eyebrow	Ceja	**SAY**-hah
Eyelash	Pestaña	pace-**TAN**-ya
Eyelid	Párpado	**PAR**-pa-doe
Pupil	Pupila	poo-**PEE**-la
Tear duct	Conducto lagrimar	con-**DUKE**-toe la-cree-**MAR**

The Body — El Cuerpo

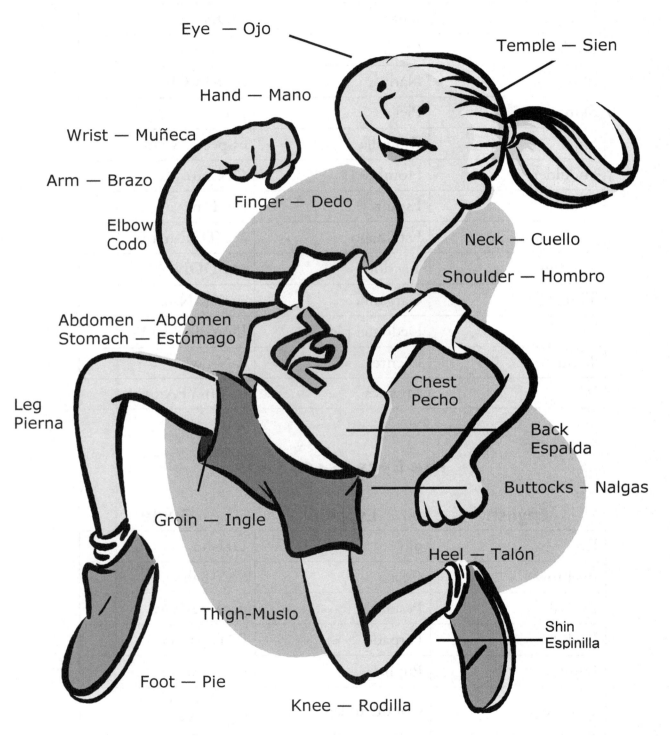

Eye — Ojo

Temple — Sien

Hand — Mano

Wrist — Muñeca

Arm — Brazo

Finger — Dedo

Elbow
Codo

Neck — Cuello

Shoulder — Hombro

Abdomen —Abdomen
Stomach — Estómago

Chest
Pecho

Leg
Pierna

Back
Espalda

Buttocks – Nalgas

Groin — Ingle

Heel — Talón

Thigh-Muslo

Shin
Espinilla

Foot — Pie

Knee — Rodilla

Toe — Dedo del pie

The Face — La Cara

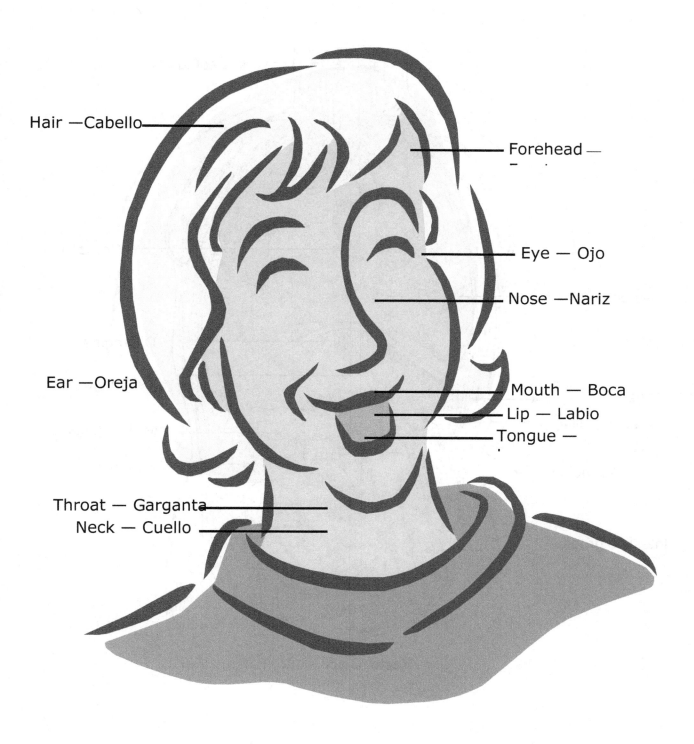

Hair —Cabello

Forehead —

Eye — Ojo

Nose —Nariz

Ear —Oreja

Mouth — Boca

Lip — Labio

Tongue —

Throat — Garganta

Neck — Cuello

Internal Organs — Órganos Internos

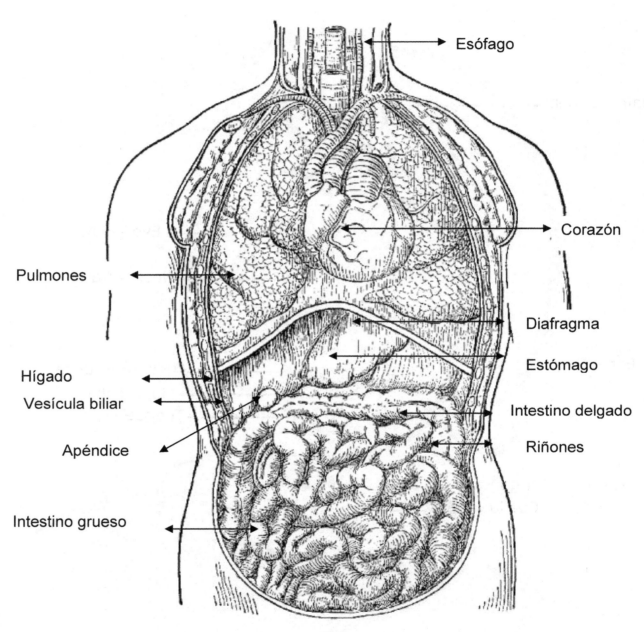

Esófago

Corazón

Pulmones

Diafragma

Estómago

Hígado

Vesícula biliar

Intestino delgado

Apéndice

Riñones

Intestino grueso

Recto, Colon, Ano

The Mouth — La Boca

English	Español	Guide
Canine	Diente canino	d-N-tay ca-**KEEN**-no
Gums	Encías	n-**SEE**-ahs
Hard palate	Paladar duro	pa-la-**DAR DO**-row
Incisor	Diente incisivo	d-**N**-tay
Molar	Muela Molar	moo-**WAY**-la no-**LAR**
Oropharynx	Orofaringe	oh-row-fa-**REEN**-hay
Soft palate	Paladar blando	pa-la-**DAR**
Teeth	Dientes	d-**N**-tays
Tongue	Lengua	**LENG**-goo-ah
Tonsil	Amígdala	ah-**MEEG**-da-la
Uvula	Úvula	**YOUVE**-oo-la

The Ear — La Oreja

English	Español	Guide
Ear canal	Conducto auditivo Canal	con-**DUKE**-toe ow-dee-**TEE**-vo ca-**NAL**
Ear drum	Tímpano	**TEEM**-pa-no
Inner ear	Oído	oh-**EE**-doe
Outer ear	Oreja	or-**RAY**-ha

Are You in Pain? — ¿Tiene Dolor?

A few years ago I was honored by being invited to attend the birth of a friend's child. "Carmen," who grew up in Puerto Rico, is fully bilingual. Spanish is her native language. She has amazing fluidity in her speech and rarely stumbles in either language. Watching the miracle of birth was amazing — but hearing the affect the physical discomfort had on Carmen's ability to speak English was even *more* eye-opening. The more pain Carmen endured, the more difficulty she had speaking and translating English. As the baby's head appeared, the three nurses who were present all said something different in English. "Push!" "She's almost here!" "It won't be long now!"

At the same time the doctor was attempting to explain to Carmen what was happening. Her sister was also in the room; she was speaking Spanish. Her husband was trying to comfort her in English. It was a cacophony! Finally, when she had had enough Carmen shouted, "Shut up! I need to hear the doctor. The rest of you just please shut up. Spanish is still my first language." When the pain increased, thinking in both languages was just too much for her.

That's when it hit me. *Even under the best conditions speaking a foreign language can be a challenge, but, when intense physical discomfort is added, the level of difficulty increases exponentially.* Pain pushes the body to its limits. Every nerve ending is working over-time. Even if they are bilingual, you must take this into consideration when working with Spanish-speaking patients. Because of the physical discomfort they are suffering, you must give them more time to translate. They are also going to have more difficulty remembering English words, *even if they've been speaking English their whole lives.*

When a Spanish-speaking patient discusses pain and discomfort, it's expressed differently than it is in English. Rather than *being* in pain, **en español** you *have* pain. Refer to the chapter on irregular verbs for more uses of **tener**. Frequently, you will hear the words *tengo dolor*, which means *I have* pain. This phrase is followed by the word for the affected area. When you are asking if the patient is in pain, use the phrase *¿tiene dolor?*

English	Español	Guide
Does it hurt?	¿Le duele?	lay do-**A**-lay
Where?	¿Dónde?	**DON**-day
Show me.	Indícalo.	een-**D**-ca-low
It hurts.	Me duele.	may do-**A**-lay
They hurt.	Me duelen	may do-**A**-lynn
Do you have pain?	¿Tiene dolor?	t-**N**-a doe-**LORE**
Do you have a lot of pain?	¿Tiene mucho dolor?	t-**N**-a **MOO**-cho doe-**LORE**
Is the pain mild?	¿Tiene dolor moderado?	t-**N**-a doe-**LORE** mo-dare-**RAH**-doe
Is the pain intermittent?	¿Tiene dolor intermitente?	t-**N**-a doe-**LORE** n-ter-me-**TENT**-tay
Is the pain deep?	¿Tiene dolor profundo?	t-**N**-a doe-**LORE** pro-**FOON**-doe
Is the pain constant?	¿Tiene dolor constante?	t-**N**-a doe-**LORE** con-**STAN**-tay
Is the pain burning?	¿Tiene dolor quemante?	t-**N**-a doe-**LORE** kay-**MAN**-tay
Is the pain severe?	¿Tiene dolor muy fuerte?	t-**N**-a doe-**LORE** foo-**AIR**-tay
Is the pain throbbing?	¿Tiene dolor pulsante?	t-**N**-a doe-**LORE** pull-**SAN**-tay
Using the numbers from one through ten indicate the level of your pain.	Usando los números de uno hasta diez, indique el nivel de su dolor.	oo-**SAND**-doe los **NEW**-may-rows day **OO**-no **AH**-sta d-**ACE** n-**D**-kay l knee-**VEL** day su do-**LORE**

Diseases — Enfermedades

In this list of common diseases, the strong relationship between our two languages is *obvio*, isn't it? Did you notice that the Spanish word "*enfermedad*" looks a lot

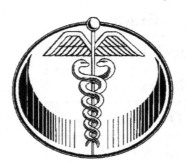

like the English word "infirmity"? It won't take you long to get the hang of this. Here's a tip to help you get started. Diseases which end in the suffix "*-itis*," like arthritis, bursitis, and tendonitis will be essentially the same words in Spanish. If the words aren't identical, try using the Latin roots from your medical studies. That's another good place to start.

English	Español	Guide
Anemia	Anemia	ah-**NAY**-me-ah
Appendicitis	Apendicitis	ah-pen-d-**SEE**-tees
Arthritis	Artritis	are-**TREE**-tees
Asthma	Asma	**AS**-ma
Bacterial infection	Infección bacteriana	een-fec-see-**ON** back-ter-ree-**AHN**-na
Bronchitis	Bronquitis	bron-**KEY**-tees
Cancer	Cáncer	**KAHN**-cer
Chicken pox	Varicela	va-ree-**SAY**-la
Cold	Catarro	ca-**TAR**-row
Diabetes	Diabetes	d-ah-**BAY**-tes
Fever	Fiebre	fee-**A**-bray
Flu	Influenza	n-flew-**N**-sa
Gall stones	Cálculos en la vesícula	**CAL**-coo-lows n la vay-**SEE**-coo-la
Glaucoma	Glaucoma	gl-ow-**CO**-ma
Hay fever	Fiebre de heno	fee-**A**-bray day **A**-no

English	Español	Guide
Hepatitis	Hepatitis	ape-ah-**T**-tis
Herpes	Herpes	**AIR**-pays
High blood pressure	Presión arterial alta	pray-see-**ON** are-tay-ree-**AL**
Hives	Urticaria	oor-t-**CA**-ree-ah
Hypoglycemia	Hipoglucemia	ee-po-glue-**SAY**-me-ah
Indigestion	Indigestión	n-dee-hess-t-**ON**
Jaundice	Ictericia	ick-tay-**REE**-see-ah
Kidney stones	Cálculos en los riñones	**CAL**-coo-lows n los reen-**NYO**-nays
Laryngitis	Laringitis	la-reen-**HE**-tees
Leukemia	Leucemia	lay-oo-**SAY**-me-ah
Measles	Sarampión	sa-ram-pee-**ON**
Mononucleosis	Mononucleosis	mo-no-new-clay-**OH**-sis
Mumps	Paperas	pa-**PEAR**-rahs
Pneumonia	Pulmonía	pool-mo-**KNEE**-ah
	Neumonía	nay-oo-mon-**KNEE**-ah
Tuberculosis	Tuberculosis	too-bear-coo-**LOW**-sis

TIPS AND TIDBITS

A six-year, federally funded project that studied the health and life span of Latinos in the United States suggested that despite having less access to healthcare and higher poverty rates, Latinos have longer life spans than other groups. The research study followed 16,000 Latinos including those of Mexican descent, Cubans, Puerto Ricans and those of Central and South American descent.

Other Common Problems

Perhaps your patient has something which is going to require further tests and treatment. Here is a list of common symptoms and conditions that you may encounter. Knowing this list of common terms will help you make a correct diagnosis *muy rápido!*

English	Español	Guide
Abscess	Absceso	ab-**SAY**-so
Blister	Ampolla	am-**PO**-ya
Broken bone	Hueso roto	who-**AY**-so **ROW**-toe
Bruise	Contusión	con-too-see-**ON**
Bump	Hinchazón	eem-cha-**SEWN**
Burn	Quemadura	kay-ma-**DO**-ra
Chills	Escalofrío	es-ca-low-**FREE**-oh
Cough	Tos	toes
Cramps	Calambre	ca-**LAMB**-bray
Diarrhea	Diarrea	dee-ah-**RAY**-ah
Fever	Fiebre	fee-**A**-bray
Hiccups	Hipo	**EE**-po
Lump	Bulto	**BOOL**-toe
Migraine	Jaqueca	ja-**KAY**-ca
	Migraña	me-**GRAN**-ya
Rash	Erupción	a-roop-see-**ON**
Sprain	Torcedura	tor-say-**DO**-ra
Swelling	Inflamación	een-fla-ma-see-**ON**
Wound	Herida	a-**REE**-da

Phrases to Describe an Illness

Yo no puedo dormir.	I can't sleep.
Yo estornudo.	I'm sneezing.
Yo estoy agotado (a).	I'm exhausted.
Yo tengo náusea.	I'm nauseous.
Me duele todo el cuerpo.	I hurt everywhere.
Yo estoy sangrando.	I'm bleeding.
Me siento mal.	I feel bad.

Remedies and Medicines
Remedios y Medicinas

You are going to be pleasantly surprised when you see all the English Spanish matches or *cognates* in this list of remedies and medicines. These really are your *amigos*! Since many drugs or *drogas* are invented in the US, often a medicine's name is derived from Latin. This gives our vocabulary substantial common ground. Even product names are good to try. *El Tylenol* is, after all a global product!

English	Español	Guide
Tablet	Tableta	ta-**BLAY**-ta
Capsule	Cápsula	**CAP**-soo-la
Pill	Píldora	**PEEL**-dor-ah
Lozenge	Pastilla	pahs-**T**-ya
Analgesic	Analgésico	ah-nal-**HEY**-see-co
Anesthetic	Anestésico	ah-nay-**STAY**-see-co
Antacid	Antiácido	ahn-t-**AH**-see-doe
Antibiotic	Antibiótico	ahn-t-b-**OH**-t-co
Anticoagulant	Anticoagulante	ahn-t-co-ah-goo-**LAN**-tay

English	Español	Guide
Antidote	Antídoto	ahn-T-oh-doe
Antihistamine	Antihistamínicos	ahn-t-ees-ta-**MEAN**-knee-cos
Anti-inflammatory	Anti-inflamatorio	ahn-t-een-fla-ma-**TOR**-ree-oh
Antiseptic	Antiséptico	ahn-t-**SEP**-t-co
Aspirin	Aspirina	ahs-p-**REE**-na
Astringent	Astringente	ah-streen-**HEN**-tay
Barbiturate	Barbitúrico	bar-b-**TOO**-ree-co
Chemotherapy	Quimioterapia	key-me-oh-ter-**RA**-p-ah
Codeine	Codeína	co-day-**EE**-na
Contraceptive	Contraceptivo	con-tra-cep-**T**-vo
Cough drop	Pastillas para la tos	pas-**T**-yas **PA**-ra la toes
Cough syrup	Jarabe para la tos	ha-**RA**-bay **PA**-ra la toes
Cortisone	Cortisona	core-tee-**SO**-na
Cream	Crema	**CRAY**-ma
Diuretic	Diurético	d-oo-**RAY**-t-co
Disinfectant	Desinfectante	des-een-fec-**TAN**-tay
Ear drops	Gotas para el oído	**GO**-tas **PA**-rah l **OH**-e-**DOE**
Eye drops	Gotas para los ojos	**GO**-tas **PA**-rah los **OH**-hos
Inhaler	Inhalador	n-ah-la-**DOOR**
Insulin	Insulina	n-soo-**LEAN**-ah
Laxative	Laxante	lax-**AN**-tay

English	Español	Guide
Liniment	Linimento	lean-knee-**MEN**-toe
Lotion	Loción	lo-see-**ON**
Morphine	Morfina	more-**FEE**-na
Narcotic	Narcótico	nar-**CO**-t-co
Nitroglycerine	Nitroglicerina	knee-tro-glee-ser-**REE**-na
Nutritional Supplement	Suplemento nutricional	sou-play-**MEN**-toe new-tree-see-on-**NAL**
Penicillin	Penicilina	pay-knee-see-**LEE**-na
Saline	Salina	sah-**LEE**-na
Sedative	Sedante	say-**DAN**-tay
Solution	Solución	so-lou-see-**ON**
Steroid	Esteroide	es-stair-**ROY**-day
Suppositories	Supositorios	sue-po-see-**TOR**-ree-ohs
Tranquilizers	Tranquilizantes	tran-key-lee-**SAN**-tays
Vaccine	Vacuna	va-**COO**-na
Vitamins	Vitaminas	v-ta-**ME**-nas

TIPS & TIDBITS

The Spanish word "*seguro*" is used in many important phrases. Even though this word actually means "insurance," it is also a part of the translation of "Social Security." In Spanish that's "*seguro social*" (say-**GOO**-row so-see-**AL**). Review the following phrases where the word "*seguro*" is used.

1. Medical insurance   Seguro medico
2. Dental insurance   Seguro dental
3. Disability insurance   Seguro de incapacidad
4. Social security   Seguro social

Side Effects — Efectos Adversos

After prescribing a medication for your patient, your next step will be to discuss possible side effects. It doesn't matter what language you speak; side effects are never pleasant. In *español* there are several ways to address the term "side effects." You can be quite literal and call them bad or adverse effects, like the title of this section demonstrates. In addition, the phrase "bad reaction" or *mala reacción* is also used.

English	Español	Guide
Allergies	Alergias	al-**LAIR**-he-ahs
Anxiety	Ansiedad	an-see-a-**DAD**
Bad reaction	Mala reacción	**MAL**-ah ray-ax-see-**ON**
Bleeding	Sangrado	san-**GRA**-doe
Constipation	Estreñimiento	es-train-knee-me-**N**-toe
Cramps	Calambres	ca-**LAMB**-rays
Decrease of appetite	Disminución del apetito	dis-me-new-see-**ON** del ah-pay-**T**-toe
Dizziness	Mareos	ma-**RAY**-ohs
	Vértigo	**VER**-t-go
Dry mouth	Boca seca	**BOW**-ca **SAY**-ca
Head ache	Dolor de cabeza	doe-**LORE** day ca-**BAY**-sa
High blood pressure	Presión alta	pray-see-**ON AL**-ta
Hives	Ronchas de la piel	**RON**-chas day la p-**L**
Increase of appetite	Aumento del apetito	ow-**MEN**-toe del ah-pay-**T**-toe
Insomnia	Insomnio	n-**SOM**-knee-oh

English	Español	Guide
Itching	Picazón	p-ca-**SEWN**
Low blood pressure	Presión arterial baja	pray-see-**ON** are-tay-ree-**AL** **BA**-ha
Photosensitivity	Sensibilidad a la luz solar	sen-see-b-lee-**DAD** ah la loose so-**LAR**
Rash	Erupción	a-rupt-see-**ON**
Sleepiness	Sueño	sue-**AY**-nyo
Tremor	Temblor	tem-**BLORE**
Weight gain	Aumento de peso	ow-**MEN**-toe day **PAY**-so

Uses and Indications — Usos y Indicaciones

If the patient is unsure why the doctor has prescribed a certain medication, you should be acquainted with the most common complains. There are lots of cognates in this list to help you explain why taking the *medicina es importante.*

English	Español	Guide
Use for	Use para	**OO**-say **PA**-rah
AIDS	SIDA	**SEE**-da
	Síndrome de inmunodeficiencia adquirida	**SEEN**-drom-a day een-moo-no-deh-fee-see-**N**-see-ah add-key-**REE**-da
Allergies	Alergias	al-**LAIR**-he-ahs

English	Español	Guide
Anxiety	Ansiedad	an-see-ay-**DAD**
Arrhythmias	Palpitaciones	pal-p-ta-see-**ON**-ace
Arthritis	Artritis	art-**REE**-tis
Asthma	Asma	**AHS**-ma
Backache	Dolor de espalda	doe-**LORE** day es-**PAL**-da
Bacteria	Bacteria	back-**TAY**-ree-ah
Bladder infection	Infección de vejiga	n-fec-see-**ON** day vay-**HE**-ga
Blood pressure	Presión arterial	pray-see-**ON** are-tay-ree-**AL**
	Presión sanguínea	pray-see-**ON** san-**GOOWE**-nay-ah
	Tensión arterial	ten-see-**ON** are-tay-ree-**AL**
Chest pain	Dolor de pecho	doe-**LORE** day **PAY**-cho
Cold (head)	Catarro	ca-**TAR**-row
Cold (chest)	Grippe	**GREE**-pay
Colic	Cólico	**CO**-lee-co
Constipation	Estreñimiento	es-train-knee-me-**N**-toe
Cough	Tos	toes
Cramps	Calambres	ca-**LAMB**-rays
Cyst	Quiste	**KEES**-tay
Depression	Depresión	day-pray-see-**ON**
Diaper rash	Exantema del pañal	x-an-**TAY**-ma del pahn-**YAL**

English	Español	Guide
Diarrhea	Diarrea	dee-ah-**RAY**-ah
Dizziness	Mareos	ma-**RAY**-os
Earache	Dolor de oído	doe-**LORE** day oh-**EE**-doe
Erectile dysfunction	Disfunción eréctil	dees-fun-see-**ON** a-**WRECK**-teal
Eczema	Eccema	a-**SAY**-ma
Fever	Fiebre	fee-**A**-bray
Fluid retention	Retención de flujo	ray-ten-see-**ON** day **FLU**-hos
Fungus	Hongo	**OWN**-go
Gout	Gota	**GO**-ta
Headache	Dolor de cabeza	doe-**LORE** day ca-**BAY**-sa
High blood pressure	Presión arterial alta	pray-see-**ON** art-tay-ree-**AL AL**-ta
HIV	VIH Virus de la inmunodeficiencia humana	vay e **AH**-chay VEE-roos day la een-moo-no-day-fee-see-**N**-see-ah oo-**MAN**-na
Hypertension	Hipotensión	e-po-ten-see-**ON**
Hyperthyroidism	Hipertiroidismo	e-pear-t-roid-**EES**-mo
Indigestion	Indigestión	een-d-hess-t-**ON**
Infection	Infección	n-fec-see-**ON**
Inflammation	Inflamación	n-flah-ma-see-**ON**
Insomnia	Insomnio	n-**SOM**-knee-oh
Lice	Piojos	pee-**OH**-hos
Menstrual pain	Dolor de la menstruación	doe-**LORE** day la men-strew-ah-see-**ON**

English	Español	Guide
Motion sickness	Mareo	ra-**RAY**-ohs
Nasal decongestant	Descongestionante nasal	day-con-hess-t-on-**NAHN**-tay na-**SAL**
Nausea	Náusea	**NOW**-see-ah
Pain	Dolor	doe-**LORE**
PMS	Síndrome premenstrual	**SEEN**-dro-may pray-men-strew-**AL**
Pregnant	Embarazada	eem-bar-rah-**SA**-da
Psoriasis	Psoriasis	see-or-**E**-ah-sis
Shortness of breath	Respiración corta	ray-spire-ah-see-**ON** **CORE**-ta
Sleep	Dormir	door-**MIR**
Sore throat	Dolor de garganta	doe-**LORE** day gar-**GAN**-ta
Stomach pain	Dolor de estómago	doe-**LORE** day ace-**TOE**-ma-go
Stress	Estrés	es-**TRES**
Stuffy nose	Nariz tupida	**NA**-reese too-**P**-da
Stye	Orzuelo	or-soo-**WAY**-low
Swelling	Hinchazón	een-cha-**SON**
Tooth ache	Dolor del diente	doe-**LORE** day dee-**N**-tay
Ulcers	Úlcera	**OOL**-sa-rah
Vomiting	Vomitando	vo-me-**TAHN**-doe
Yeast infection	Infección de levadura	een-fec-see-**ON** day lay-va-**DOO**-rah

TIPS AND TIDBITS

La familia is the soul of Latino culture. The family also plays a very important role in healthcare decisions. Often patients will seek the recommendations of family members when selecting a doctor or a hospital. Everyone's opinion is considered and carefully weighed. In addition, if a family member is diagnosed with an illness that requires a life-style change, like diet modification, he or she may choose not to follow the healthcare provider's recommendations the changes are deemed to be too difficult for the family. As you treat Spanish-speaking patients, don't forget that you are essentially treating the entire family!

Refills — Rellenos

Drugs and their administration vary widely from country to country. Your Spanish-speaking patients may look for medications in local markets that require a prescription in the US. Many Latinos don't understand why a drug which can be purchased over the counter in their country of origin requires a prescription here. Several countries even allow patients to administer their own injections particularly of antibiotics. To complicate matters even further, Latin America has a strong history of non-traditional medicine including herbs and homeopathic remedies.

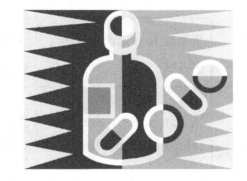

Frequently patients will try a variety of home remedies, before visiting the pharmacy, doctor's office or hospital.

English	Español	Guide
No refills	No hay rellenos	no ay ray-YEA-nose
	No hay repeticiones	no eye ray-pay-t-see-ON-ace
	No se puede repetir	no say poo-A-day ray-pay-TEAR

83

English	Español	Guide
Do you need a refill?	¿Necesita un relleno?	nay-say-**SEE**-ta oon ray-**YEA**-no
You may repeat this once.	Se puede repetir esta una vez.	say poo-**A**-day ray-pay-**TEAR ACE**-ta **OO**-na vase
You may repeat this prescription # times.	Se puede repetir esta receta médica # veces.	say poo-**A**-day ray-pay-**TEAR ACE**-ta ray-**SAY**-ta **MAY**-dee-ca # **VASE**-ace
Please contact your doctor.	Favor de consultar a su doctor.	fa-**VOR** day con-sool-**TAR** ah sue doc-**TOR**
Your doctor changed your prescription.	Su doctor se cambió su receta médica.	sue doc-**TOR** say cam-b-**OH** sue ray-say-**TA MAY**-dee-ca
What is your doctor's name?	¿Cuál es el nombre de su doctor?	coo-**ALL** ace L **NOM**-bray day sue doc-**TOR**
What is your doctor's telephone number?	¿Cuál es el número de teléfono de su doctor?	coo-**ALL** ace L **NEW**-may-row day tay-**LAY**-fono day sue doc-**TOR**
Please wait.	Favor de esperar.	fa-**VOR** day es-pay-**RARE**
I am going to call your doctor.	Voy a llamar a su doctor.	voy ah ya-**MAR** ah sue doc-**TOR**
I am going to call your doctor for authorization to renew your prescription.	Voy a llamar a su doctor para que autorice la repetición de su receta médica.	voy ah ya-**MARE** ah sue doc-**TOR PA**-ra kay ow-toe-**REE**-say la ray-pay-t-see-**ON** de sue ray-**SAY**-ta **MAY**-dee-ca

English	Español	Guide
Are you using over the counter medications?	¿Usa medicinas sin receta médica?	OO-sa may-dee-SEEN-ah seen ray-SAY-ta MAY-dee-ca
Are you using herbal products?	¿Usa productos naturales o remedios caseros?	OO-sa pro-DUKE-toes na-too-RA-lace oh
Are you using home remedies?	¿Usa remedios caseros?	OO-sa ray-MAY-dee-ohs ca-SAY-rows

Dispensing Instructions—Las Instrucciones

Here's an important tip on your choice of phrases to you when you are double-checking to make sure that your Spanish-speaking patient has understood the instructions you have given them pertaining to a medication. In this situation always use the phrase "do you understand my instructions." This is much better than asking "do you understand my directions." If you think back to some of the important question phrases you learned earlier, you will remember that a *dirección* in *español* is an address. Using this word could confuse someone who is learning to speak English. The word instruction in English is *instrucción* in Spanish. There's no confusion there!

English	Español	Guide
Prescription	Receta médica	ray-SAY-ta MAY-d-ka
	Fórmula	FOR-moo-la
	Receta	ray-SAY-ta

English	Español	Guide
Take the medicine	Toma la medicina	**TOE**-ma la may-d-**SEEN**-na
Before meals	Antes de las comidas	**AN**-tays day las co-**ME**-das
Between meals	Entre las comidas	**N**-tray las co-**ME**-das
After meals	Después de las comidas	days-poo-**ACE** day las co-**ME**-das
In the morning	Por la mañana	pour la man-**YA**-na
In the afternoon	Por la tarde	pour la **TAR**-day
In the evening	Por la noche	pour la **NO**-chay
At bedtime	A la hora de acostarse	ah la **OR**-ah day ah-co-**STAR**-say
Only when you have pain	Solo cuando tiene dolor	**SO**-low coo-**AN**-doe t-**N**-a doe-**LORE**
As directed by your doctor	Según las instrucciones de su doctor.	say-**GOON** las n-strook-see-**ON**-ace day sue doc-**TOR**
With water	Con agua	con **AH**-goo-ah
With milk	Con leche	con **LAY**-chay
With food	Con la comida	con la co-**ME**-da
With breakfast	Con el desayuno	con L day-say-**OO**-no
With lunch	Con el almuerzo	con L al-moo-**AIR**-so
With dinner	Con la cena	con la **SAY**-na
On an empty stomach	Con el estómago vacío.	con l ace-**TOE**-ma-go va-**SEE**-oh
Only when necessary	Solo cuando es necesario	**SO**-low coo-**AN**-doe es nay-say-**SAR**-ree-oh

English	Español	Guide
Take the medicine # times per day.	Toma la medicina # veces por día.	TOE-ma la may-d-SEEN-na # VASE-aces pour D-ah
Don't swallow	No traiga	no TRY-ga
Gargle	Hace gárgaras	AH-say GAR-gar-as
Spit	Escupe	es-COO-pay
Spray	Rociada	row-see-AH-da
Syringe	Jeringuilla	hey-reen-GEE-ya

How Much and How Often — Cuánto y Cuándo

Explaining how much medicine to take and how often to take it can be extremely confusing to many patients. This requires extra care and patience. It could also call for more creativity than you are accustomed to using with your English-speaking patients. Some healthcare providers become extremely resourceful in getting the information across. Draw pictures if you must in order to communicate. In some areas where patients have trouble reading, some healthcare professionals create drawings of a sunrise, noonday sun, and moon to represent three times per day, morning, noon, and night.

It's a simple strategy and an effective one. Isn't it a good thing that the number three always looks like a three whether you speak English or Spanish?

How Much	¿Cuánto?	coo-WAN-toe
English	**Español**	**Guide**
Take	Toma	TOE-ma
A cup	Una copa	OO-na CO-pa

English	Español	Guide
A drop	Una gota	**OO**-na **GO**-ta
A glass	Un vaso	**OON VA**-so
Apply	Aplique	ah-**PLEA**-kay
Bottle	Botella	bow-**TAY**-ya
By mouth	Por boca	pour **BOW**-ca
Dropper	Cuentagotas	coo-**WAYNE**-ta **GO**-tas
Externally	Externamente	x-ter-na-**MEN**-tay
For external use	Para uso externo	**PA**-ra **OO**-so x-**TER**-no
Half	Una media	**OO**-na may-**D**-ah
Inhale	Inhale	een-**AH**-lay
Injection	Inyección	een-yeck-see-**ON**
Insert	Inserta	een-**SER**-ta
Keep refrigerated	Guarda en el refrigerador	goo-**WAHR**-da in l ray-free-hair-ray-**DOOR**
Label	Etiqueta	a-tee **KAY**-ta
Milliliter	Mililitro	me-lee-**LEE**-tro
Mix	Mezclar	mace-**CLAR**
One drop	Una gota	**OO**-na **GO**-ta
One half teaspoon	Una media cucharadita	**OO**-na may-**D**-ah coo-char-ra-**D**-ta
One quarter	Un cuarto	oon coo-**ARE**-toe
One tablespoon	Una cucharada	**OO**-na coo-char-**RA**-da
One teaspoon	Una cucharadita	**OO**-na coo-char-ra-**D**-ta

English	Español	Guide
One third	Un tercero	oon ter-**SAY**-row
Patch	Parche	**PAR**-chay
Rectal Suppository	Supositorio rectal	sue-po-see-**TOR**-ree-oh wreck-**TAL**
Safety cap	Tapón de seguridad	ta-**PON** day say-goo-ree-**DAD**
Shake well	Agítese bien	ah-**HE**-tay-say b-n
Sparingly	Poco	**PO**-co
Swallow	Traiga	**TRYEYE**-ga
Swish	Susurro	sue-**SEWER**-oh
To affected areas	En las áreas afectadas	N las **AH**-ray-as ah-fec-**TA**-das
Unwrap	Desempaqueta	des-m-pa-**KAY**-ta
Vaginal Suppository	Supositorio vaginal	sue-po-see-**TOR**-ree-oh va-he-**NAL**
Vapor nebulizer	Nebulizador de vapor	nay-boo-lee-sa-**DOOR** day va-**POUR**
Vial	Vial	vee-**AHL**
Z-Pack: Take 2 tablets by mouth today. Then take one tablet each day for 4 more days.	Toma dos tabletas por boca hoy. Entonces toma una tableta por boca cada día para cuatro días más.	**TOE**-ma dose ta-**BLAY**-tas pour **BOW**-ca oy. n-**TONE**-says **TOE**-ma **OO**-na ta-**BLAY**-ta pour **BOW**-ca **CA**-da **D**-ah **PA**-rah coo-**AH**-tro **D**-ahs mas

When   Cuándo

English	Español	Guide
Take _____ times	Toma _____ veces	TOE-ma _____ VAY-says
Every day	Cada día	CA-da DEE-ah
Until finished	Hasta que se termina	AH-sta kay say ter-ME-na
Every ____ hours	Cada _____ horas	CA-da _____ OR-ahs
_____ times per day	_____ veces al día	_____ VAY-says al DEE-ah
For _____ days	Por _____ días	Pour _____ DEE-ahs
For _____ weeks	Por _____ semanas	Pour _____ say-MAN-nas
For _____ months	Por _____ meses	Pour _____ MAY-says

TIPS & TIDBITS

Because it can have dangerous side effects, **Dyperone** was taken off the US market in the late 1970s It is still available today in Mexico. Going by the street name *"Aspirina Mexicana,"* it can be purchased over the counter in many Hispanic-owned convenience stores across the country.

Calming Customers — Calmando Clientes

Building a good relationship with Latino customers is what good customer service is all about. The path to starting that relationship often begins with a smile and a simple phrase or two. On the following list you will find some great "one-liners" that will help you get started. Talking to parents about their children is a great way to begin. Practice these often and have fun! You should get lots of smiles and encouragement from everyone!

English	Español	Guide
Don't worry.	No se preocupe.	no say pray-oh-**COO**-pay
Good luck!	¡Buena suerte!	boo-**WAY**-na **SWEAR**-tay
Calm down	¡Cálmese!	**CAL**-may-say
How pretty!	¡Qué bonito! (m)	kay bow-**KNEE**-toe
	¡Qué bonita! (f)	kay bow-**KNEE**-ta
	¡Qué lindo! (m)	kay **LEAN**-doe
	¡Qué linda! (f)	kay **LEAN**-da
He's precious! She's precious!	¡Es precioso!	es pray-see-**OH**-so
	¡Es preciosa!	es pray-see-**OH**-sa
What a smile!	¡Qué sonrisa!	kay son-**REE**-sa
Have a nice day!	¡Qué le vaya bien!	kay lay **VA**-ya b-**N**
	Tenga un buen día.	**TEN**-ga oon boo-**WAYNE** **DEE**-ah
How old is your baby?	¿Cuántos años tiene su bebé?	coo-**AN**-toes **AN**-yos t-**N**-a sue bay-**BAY**
What's your baby's name?	¿Cómo se llama su bebé?	**CO**-mo say **YA**-ma sue bay-**BAY**

TIPS AND TECHNIQUES

Hispanic attitudes on healthcare and medical treatment are as complex as Hispanics are themselves. By far, the largest obstacle to providing excellent healthcare services to Latinos in the US is overcoming the language barrier. However, other serious issues must be considered. For first generation Latinos attitudes about our healthcare system can also be shaped by acculturation, immigration status, level of income and previous experience with healthcare professionals.

In the Retail Store

Often customers with limited English proficiency receive poor customer in retail situations. Sometimes employees can be rude, speak too quickly, and trying to be understood, shout at the customer. The loyalty of Latin American customers is well known. Here are a variety of phrases that will help you provide great customer service.

English	Español	Guide
Please wait.	Favor de esperar.	fa-**VOR** day es-pay-**RAR**
May I help you?	¿Puedo servirle?	poo-**A**-doe sear-**VEER**-lay
One moment please	Un momento, por favor	oon mo-**MEN**-toe, pour fa-**VOR**
Please hold a moment.	Favor de esperar un momento.	fa-**VOR** day es-pay-**RAR** oon mo-**MEN**-toe
I'm going to look for a translator.	Voy a buscar un traductor.	voy ah boos-**CAR** oon tra-duke-**TOR**
Would you like to wait for your prescription?	¿Le gusta esperar para su receta médica?	lay **GOOSE**-ta es-pay-**RAR** sue ray-**SAY**-ta **MAY**-d-ca
Please sit over there.	Favor de sentarse allá.	fa-**VOR** day sen-**TAR**-say ah-**KEY**
It will take # minutes to prepare.	Necesito # minutos preparla.	nay-say-**SEE**-toe # me-**NEW**-toes pre-par-**RAR**-la

English	Español	Guide
Thank you for waiting.	Gracias para esperando.	**GRA**-see-ahs **PA**-rah es-pear-**RAR**
Your prescription will be ready this afternoon.	Su receta médica estará lista esta tarde.	sue ray-**SAY**-ta **MAY**-d-ca es-tar-**AH LEES**-ta **ACE**-ta **TAR**-day
Your prescription will be ready tomorrow.	Su receta médica estará lista mañana.	sue ray-**SAY**-ta **MAY**-d-ca es-tar-**AH LEES**-ta mahn-**YAN**-na
I'm sorry.	Lo siento	low see-**N**-toe
Your total is # dollars.	Su cuenta está # dólares.	sue coo-**AINT**-ta ace-**TA** $ **DOE**-lar-ace
Do you have insurance for your medication?	¿Tiene seguro para su medicina?	t-**N**-a say-**GOO**-row **PA**-rah sue may-dee-**SEEN**-na
I need your insurance card, please.	Necesito su tarjeta de seguro, por favor.	nay-say-see-toe sue tar-**HEY**-ta day say-**GOO**-row pour fa-**VOR**
Please sign here.	Favor de firmar aquí.	fa-**VOR** day fear-**MAR** ah-**KEY**
Come back soon.	Regrese pronto.	ray-**GRES**-a **PRON**-toe
We'll see you.	Nos vemos.	nos **VAY**-mos
Have a nice day.	¿Qué le vaya bien!	kay lay **VAI**-ya bN
We appreciate your business.	Apreciamos su negocio.	ah-pray-see-**AH**-mos sue may-**GO**-see-oh

Diabetes and Latinos

According to the American Diabetes Association, diabetes in the US Hispanic population is at epidemic proportions. Within this diverse ethnic group, diabetes is 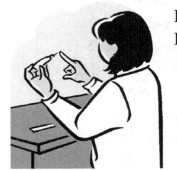 two to three times more common in Mexican American and Puerto Rican adults than it is in Central American Hispanics and Cubans. Many go undiagnosed because Hispanics have a lower than average level of preventative healthcare. It's possible that as many as 675,000 Hispanic Americans have diabetes and do not realize it. Many studies find that almost every Latino knows at least one other Latino who is affected with this disease.

English	Español	Guide
Abdomen	Abdomen	ab-**DOE**-men
Abnormal	Anormal	ah-nor-**MAL**
Ampule	Ampolleta	am-po-**YEA**-ta
Arms	Brazos	**BRA**-sos
Blood	Sangre	**SAHN**-grey
Blood sugar	Glucosa en la sangre	glue-**CO**-sa in la **SAHN**-grey
Carbohydrates	Carbohidratos	car-bow-heed-**RAH**-toes
Condition	Condición	con-d-see-**ON**
Diabetes	Diabetes	d-ah-**BET**-tays
Diabetic	Diabético *(a)*	d-a-**BET**-t-co
Dizziness	Mareos	ma-**RAY**-ohs
Dosage	Dosis	**DOE**-cease
Drop	Gota	**GO**-ta

English	Español	Guide
Energy	Energía	n-nair-**HE**-ah
Excessive	Excesivo (a)	x-ces-**SEE**-vo
Exercise	Ejercicio	a-hair-**SEE**-see-oh
Expiration date	Fecha de expiración	**FAY**-cha day x-pier-rah-see-**ON**
Fast acting	Acción rápida	ax-see-**ON** **RAH**-p-da
Fruit juice	Jugo de frutas	**WHO**-go day **FRU**-tas
Glucometer	Glucómetro	glue-**CO**-may-tro
Glucose	Glucosa	glue-**CO**-sa
Hemoglobin	Hemoglobina	e-mo-glow-**B**-na
High	Alto *(a)*	**AL**-toe
Hyperglycemia	Hiperglicemia	e-pear-glee-**SAY**-me-ah
Hypoglycemia	Hipoglicemia	e-po- glee-**SAY**-me-ah
Injection	Inyección	een-yeck-see-**ON**
Insulin	Insulina	een-sue-**LEE**-na
Intermediate acting	Acción intermedia	ax-see-**ON** een-ter-**MAY**-d-ah
Ketoacidosis	Quetoacidosis	kay-toe-ah-see-**DOSE**-cease
Ketone	Quejona	kay-**HOE**-na
Lancet	Lanceta	lan-**SAY**-ta
Level	Nivel	knee-**VEL**
Long lasting	Dura mucho tiempo	**DO**-rah **MOO**-cho t-**M**-po
Low	Bajo *(a)*	**BA**-ho

English	Español	Guide
Monitor	Monitor	mo-knee-**TOR**
Needles	Agujas	ah-**GOO**-has
Normal	Normal	nor-**MAL**
NPH insulin	Insulina NPH	een-sue-**LEE**-na N-nay-pay-**AH**-chay
Overweight	Sobrepeso	**SO**-bray-**PAY**-so
Pancreas	Páncreas	**PAHN**-cray-ahs
Premixed insulin	Insulina premezclada	een-sue-**LEE**-na pray-mess-**CLA**-da
Quantity	Cantidad	can-t-**DAHD**
Refrigerator	Refrigerador	ray-free-hair-rah-**DOOR**
Regular insulin	Insulina regular	een-sue-**LEE**-na ray-goo-**LAR**
Resistance	Resistencia	ray-cease-**TEN**-see-ah
Risk	Riesgo	ree-**ACE**-go
Snack	Merienda	may-ree-**N**-da
Sugar	Azúcar	ah-**SUE**-car
Sweats	Sudores	sue-**DOOR**-race
Syringe	Jeringuilla	hair-ring-**GEE**-ya
Therapy	Terapia	ter-**RAH**-p-ah
Thighs	Muslos	**MOOS**-lows
To control	Controlar	con-trol-**ARE**
To measure	Medir	may-**DEER**
Type 2	Tipo dos	T-po dose
Type one	Tipo uno	T-po **OO**-no
Weakness	Debilidad	day-bee-lee-**DAHD**

Common Symptoms of Diabetes

English	Español	Guide
Symptoms	Síntomas	**SEEN**-toe-mas
Chronic fatigue	Cansancio crónico	cahn-**SAHN**-see-oh **CROW**-knee-co
Thirst	Sed	said
Frequent urination	Orina con frecuencia	or-**REE**-na con fray-coo-**N**-see-ah
Blurred vision	Visión borrosa	v-see-**ON** bow-**ROW**-sa
Sudden weight loss	Pérdida súbita de peso	**PEAR**-d-da **SUE**-b-ta day **PAY**-so
Sexual problems	Problemas sexuales	pro-**BLAY**-mas sex-oo-**AL**-ace
Wounds that won't heal	Heridas que no sanan	air-**REE**-das kay no **SA**-nan
Vaginal infections	Infecciones vaginales	een-fec-see-**ON**-ace va-he-**NAL**-ace
Numbness or tingling in the hands or feet	Adormecimiento u hormigueo en las manos o pies	ah-door-may-see-me-**N**-toe oo or-me-**GWAY**-nay-oh in las **MA**-nose oh p-**ACE**

Diet, Cuisine and Nutritional Counseling

Foods and cuisine in Latin America are as diverse as the people are. Principally, meals are based on typical products found in each country or region. When Americans think about Latin American foods, many think mostly of Mexican food, but there is a wider diversity of tastes and dishes than that! What we consider to be Mexican food is actually more of a "Tex-Mex" style of cooking. A more traditional Mexican diet is often composed of pre-Colombian, French and Spanish dishes. It's also important to consider that the foods and spices used in Mexico are quite different from those used in Central or South American cooking. Listed below are some common factors found in many Latin American diets:

- ✓ Most breads are based on corn rather than wheat.

- ✓ Beans are a common source of protein. Many countries favor one type of bean over another. For example, black beans are associated with Cuba, pinto beans are associated with Mexico, and pink beans are a favorite in Puerto Rico.

- ✓ Rice is more commonly consumed than potatoes.

- ✓ Beef ranks high with Hispanics in terms of taste and prestige. Chicken is viewed as being healthier than either pork or beef, and among some groups seafood is the most popular meat.

- ✓ Latinos tend to seek brand names for assurances of nutrition and quality.

- ✓ Hispanics have a higher than average fat intake and a lower consumption of dairy products, fruits and vegetables.

- ✓ High prevalence of obesity. Carrying some "weight" is often seen as being well off and healthy, indicating income and success.

- ✓ Many Latinos hold healthcare professionals in high regard.

- ✓ Treat your Latin American clients with the utmost courtesy and respect.

- ✓ Use surnames and titles (Señor, Señora, and Señorita) at your first meeting. For younger Latinos proceed carefully with first names after you feel that you have established rapport. With older Latin Americans, *always* use courtesy titles.

- ✓ Ask about the language spoken in the home. Latinos can be completely bilingual, speak some English, or speak no English at all. Don't assume that because a person speaks Spanish that they are able to read or write in Spanish.

✓ Learn about new fruits and vegetables that are a part of Latin American diets like yucca and plantains.

✓ Gain the support of family members in your care plan — especially those members of the family that do the shopping and prepare the food. They are your best allies in changing bad nutritional habits.

✓ Latin Americans are extremely diverse. Identifying your client's cultural background will also give you clues into meal patterns and preferences.

✓ Determine the level of your client's acculturation. More acculturated individuals are usually more flexible in trying new foods.

✓ The traditional Latin American diet is high in fiber and relies mainly on vegetable protein. Use this to your advantage!

HIV and AIDS Counseling

The HIV/AIDS epidemic is an extremely serious threat to the nation's Hispanic community. In addition to being a population that is seriously affected by HIV, Latinos continue to face serious challenges in accessing healthcare, prevention services, and treatment. In 2001 HIV/AIDS was the third leading cause of death among Hispanic men aged 35-44. It was the fourth leading cause of death among Hispanic women in the same age group.

Although Hispanics make up only about 14% of the total US population, they account for 18% or almost 164,000 of the more than 886,500 AIDS cases diagnosed since the beginning of the epidemic twenty-five years ago. It's estimated that by the end of 2002, nearly 88,000 Hispanics had died with AIDS.

When you are trying to explain sensitive material involving sex and sexual conduct to Spanish-speaking clients, always remember to go very slowly. This is especially important with language barriers present challenges to communication. Matters involving sex and sexual conduct are delicate and difficult to discuss, even when everyone speaks the same language. The following key words and phrases will help you. Start slowly and focus on learning only 10 words. Go over the list with a highlighter and highlight the 10 that you will use most often. Learn them first. When you've mastered those, go on to 10 more words. If you work with small portions of vocabulary, you will not let the learning process overwhelm you.

English	Español	Guide
HIV	VIH Virus de la inmunodeficiencia humana	vay e **AH**-chay **VEE**-roos day la een-moo-no-day-fee-see-**N**-see-ah oo-**MAN**-na
AIDS	SIDA Síndrome de inmunodeficiencia adquirida	**SEE**-da **SEEN**-drom-a day een-moo-no-day-fee-see-**N**-see-ah add-key-**REE**-da
Abscess	Absceso	ab-**SAY**-so
Anus	Ano	**AH**-no
Blister	Ampollas	am-**PO**-yas
Blood	Sangre	**SAHN**-grey
Condom	Condón	con-**DOHN**
Contact	Contacto	con-**TAC**-toe
Fluids	Fluidos	flu-**E**-dos
Immune system	Sistema inmunitario	sis-**TAY**-ma een-moon-knee-**TAR**-e-oh
Oral sex	Sexo oral	**SEX**-oh or-**AL**
Penis	Pene	**PAY**-nay

English	Español	Guide
Protection	Protección	pro-tec-see-**ON**
Rash	Erupción	a-rupe-see-**ON**
Rectum	Recto	**WRECK**-toe
Risk	Riesgo	ree-**ACE**-go
Semen	Semen	say-**MEN**
Sex	Sexo	**SEX**-oh
Sexual relations	Coito sexual	co-**E**-to sex-oo-**AL**
Swelling	Hinchazón	een-cha-**SEWN**
Syringes	Jeringas	hair-**RING**-gas
To prevent	Prevenir	pray-ven-**NEAR**
Transmission	Transmisión	trans-me-see-**ON**
Urine	Orina	or-**REEN**-na
Vagina	Vagina	va-**HE**-na
Virus	Virus	**VEE**-russ
Without protection	Sin protección	seen Pro-tec-see-**ON**

TIPS AND TIDBITS

A variety of public service ads are commonly seen on Spanish language television stations warning viewers about the dangers of AIDS and HIV. Themes on these public service announcements cover the risks of having unprotected sex and raise awareness about the disease in the US. In the TV ads AIDS is translated with the acronym "**SIDA**" (SEE-da). It's one of the few terms in Spanish that is shortened to an acronym rather than being stated fully word for word. Everyone who speaks Spanish understands the term SIDA.

Para Practicar

In the space provided, use the following common medications and write the appropriate dispensing instructions in Spanish. Use these pages as a quick reference guide— and add to the list of medications as you continue to study the patients in the communities you serve. The following website provided by the National Institute of Health can help you. It lists the most commonly dispensed medications in Spanish along with drug interaction and side effects. This is a great website for expanding your knowledge and vocabulary!

www.nlm.nih.gov/medlineplus/spanish/druginformation.html

Ambien_____

_____

_____

_____

Aspirin_____

_____

_____

_____

Amoxicillin

_____

_____

_____

_____

Coumadin_____

_____

_____

_____

Digoxin_____

_____

_____

_____

Dilantin_____

_____

_____

_____

Effexor_____

_____

_____

_____

Fluvastatin_____

_____

_____

_____

Gentamycin_____

_____

_____

_____

Heparin_____

_____

_____

_____

Ibuprofen_____

_____

_____

_____

Insulin_____

_____

_____

_____

Lunesta_____

_____

_____

_____

Methotrexate_____

_____

_____

_____

Niacin_____

_____

_____

_____

Prednisone_____

_____

_____

_____

Prozac_____

_____

_____

_____

Xanax_____

_____

_____

_____

One for the Road: Phrases to Use Any Time

Obviously, conversation is made up of more than just lists of words. It will take practice and determination for you to achieve free-flowing conversation in a language that's new to you. Learning Spanish is a slow and steady process for adults. It could take several months before you begin to "think" in Spanish, so don't expect to achieve native speaker speed overnight. There will be times when you feel like you can't remember anything you've studied. That's natural. It happens to everyone. Try not to be discouraged. The rewards you'll receive from learning to speak Spanish are far greater than a little bit of frustration. If you keep working, it won't be long before you'll have a breakthrough. Learning Spanish is a lot like eating a great steak. You don't want to rush it. Cut each bite of your Spanish, chew it over carefully and savor each morsel. Moving along at a slower pace will help you retain what you learn longer.

Spanish is a language that has loads of zest and flair. It is punctuated with single words and short phrases that can really express a lot of sentiment. The next time you have an opportunity to observe native speakers, listen carefully. You may hear them switch from English to Spanish, depending on what they are saying. And, you might hear them use any of the "one-liners" listed below. Phrases like these add spice to your conversation. Use the following list to help you take your conversational skills to the next level.

English	Español	Guide
Are you sure?	¿Está seguro? (a)	es-**TA** say-**GOO**-row
Excellent!	¡Excelente!	x-say-**LENT**-tay
Fantastic!	¡Fantástico!	fan-**TA**-stee-co
Good idea.	Buena idea.	boo-**A**-na e-**DAY**-ah
Happy birthday!	¡Feliz cumpleaños!	fay-**LEASE** coom-play-**AHN**-yos

English	Español	Guide
Have a nice day.	Tenga un buen día.	TEN-ga un boo-WAYNE DEE-ah
I agree.	De acuerdo.	day ah-coo-AIR-doe
I believe so.	Creo que sí.	CRAY-oh kay SEE
I'm so glad.	Me alegro.	may ah-LAY-gro
I'll be right back.	¡Ahora vengo!	ah-OR-ah VEIN-go
I'm leaving now.	¡Ya me voy!	ya may VOY
That's OK.	Está bien.	es-TA b-N
It's important.	Es importante.	es eem-pour-TAHN-tay
It's serious.	Es grave.	es GRA-vay
It's possible.	Es posible	es po-SEE-blay
Maybe.	Quizás.	key-SAHS
Me, neither	Yo tampoco.	yo tam-PO-co
Me, too	Yo también.	yo tam-b-N
More or less	Más o menos.	mas oh MAY-nos
Really?	¿De veras?	day VER-ahs
Sure	¡Claro!	CLA-row
That depends.	Depende.	day-PEN-day
We'll see you.	Nos vemos.	nos VAY-mos

TIPS & TIDBITS

Use short phrases to spice up your conversation. Start with one new phrase each week and see how many different situations you can occur where you can use your "phrase of the week."

Typing in Spanish on Your Computer
Inserting Letters with Shortcut Keys

When you need to type letters with accent marks or use Spanish punctuation, you will use keys that you have probably never used before! Actually, you are *composing characters* using the **control** key. It is located on the bottom row of keys. You will see that it is such an important key that there is one on both sides. It keeps the computer from moving forward one space so that the accent goes on *top* of the letter instead of *beside* it.

Always remember to hold the control key down first. It will be the *key* to your success in word processing Spanish. With a little practice these keys will become a normal part of your word processing skills.

Also, if using MS Word, you may use the menu command Insert>Symbol.

To insert	For a PC, Press	For a Mac, Press
á, é, í, ó, ú, ý Á, É, Í, Ó, Ú, Ý	CTRL+' (APOSTROPHE), *the letter*	OPTION + e, *the letter*
â, ê, î, ô, û Â, Ê, Î, Ô, Û	CTRL+SHIFT+^ (CARET), *the letter*	OPTION + i, *the letter*
ã, ñ, õ Ã, Ñ, Õ	CTRL+SHIFT+~ (TILDE), *the letter*	OPTION + n, *the letter*
ä, ë, ï, ö, ü, ÿ Ä, Ë, Ï, Ö, Ü, Ÿ	CTRL+SHIFT+: (COLON), *the letter*	OPTION + u, *the letter*
¿	ALT+CTRL+SHIFT+?	OPTION+SHIFT+ ?
¡	ALT+CTRL+SHIFT+!	OPTION + !

Basic Information
Please print

Date: _____
Month   Day   Year

Mr.
Mrs.
Miss_____
First Name   Middle Name   Paternal Surname   Maternal Surname   (Husband)

Address:_____
Street

_____
City   *State*   *Zip Code*

Telephone: Home_____   **Work**_____

                Cell_____   **Fax** _____

Email Address: _____

Social Security Number: _____-_____-_____

Date of birth _____
                   Month   Day   Year

Driver's License Number: _____

Occupation: _____

Place of employment: _____

Marital Status: Married
                            Single
                            Divorced
                            Separated
                            Widow

Husband's name:_____
                   First Name   Middle Name   Paternal Surname   Maternal Surname   (Husband)
Wife's name: _____
                 First Name   Middle Name   Paternal Surname Maternal Surname   (Husband)

In case of emergency: _____   **Telephone:** _____

Signature: _____   **Date:** _____

Practicing What You Have Learned

Practice is an important part of the language learning process. The more you include practice in your daily routine, the more comfortable and fluent you will become. There is no easy way to practice. It just takes time. The key to practicing Spanish is to set realistic goals. Don't let the language learning process become overwhelming to you. Yes, there is a lot to learn, and it will take some time. But, by setting realistic goals, you have a greater chance of sticking with it. Each of us have different learning styles, so find out what works best for you and break the material down into small pieces. Some of us learn best by listening. Others need to write the words and phrases in order to visualize them. Generally the more of your senses that you involve in the learning process, the faster you will retain the information. So, focus and practice one thing at a time. It's doing the little things that will make the greatest difference in the long run. Working five minutes every day on your Spanish is *mucho* better than trying to put in an hour of practice time only once each week. Consistency in your practice is critical.

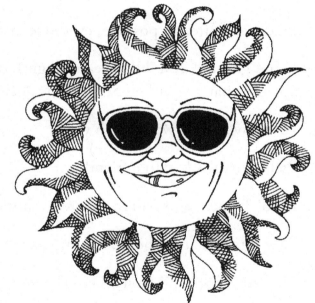

Here are some practice tips that have worked for me and others who have participated in *SpeakEasy's Survival Spanish*™ training programs over the last few years.

1. Start practicing first thing in the morning. The shower is a great place to start. Say the numbers or run through the months of the year while you wash your hair. If you practice when you start your day you are more likely to continue to practice as the day progresses.

2. Use your commute time to practice. Listening to CDs, music and Spanish language radio stations will help you get the rhythm of Spanish. It will also increase your vocabulary.

3. If you are stopped in traffic, look around you for numbers on billboards or the license tags of the cars in front of you to help you practice. Don't just sit there—do something!

4. Investigate sites on the internet. Sites such as www.about.spanish.com and www.studyspanish.com are great places to practice and to learn, not to mention the fact that they are free!

5. Buy Spanish magazines or pick up Spanish newspapers that are published in your area. Many magazines like *People* have Spanish versions and almost every community in the country has a Spanish language newspaper or two. Many of them are free.

6. If there aren't any Spanish newspapers in your area, you can find a variety of publications from Latin America online. Major cities in Latin America all have newspapers that are easy to find on-line.

7. Practice as often as possible, even five minutes a day will help.

8. Don't give up! You didn't learn English overnight and you won't learn Spanish that way either. Set realistic goals and don't go too far too fast.

9. Learn five to ten words each week.

10. Practice at work with a friend.

11. Read! These books will make great additions to your library.

Baez, Francia and Chong, Nilda. *Latino Culture*. Intercultural Press, 2005

Einsohn, Marc and Steil, Gail. *The Idiot's Guide to Learning Spanish on Your Own*. Alpha Books, 1996

Hawson, Steven R. *Learn Spanish the Lazy Way*. Alpha Books, 1999.

Reid, Elizabeth. Spanish *Lingo for the Savvy Gringo*. In One Ear Publications, 1997

Wald, Susana. *Spanish for Dummies*. Wiley Publishing, 2000.

About the Author

Myelita Melton, MA

Myelita Melton, founder of SpeakEasy Communications, remembers the first time she heard a "foreign" language. She knew from that moment what she wanted to do with her life. "Since I was always the kid in class that talked too much," Myelitia says, "I figured it would be a good idea to learn more than one language-that way I could talk to a lot more people!" After high school, she studied in Mexico at the *Instituto de Filológica Hispánica* and completed both her BA and MA in French and Curriculum Design at Appalachian State University in Boone, NC. She has studied five languages: French, Spanish, Italian, German, and English.

"Lita's" unique career includes classroom instruction and challenging corporate experience. She has won several national awards, including a prestigious *Rockefeller* scholarship. In 1994 she was named to *Who's Who Among Outstanding Americans*. Myelita's corporate experience includes owning a television production firm, working with NBC's Spanish news division, *Canal de Noticias,* and Charlotte's PBS affiliate WTVI. In her spare time, she continues to broadcast with WDAV, a National Public Radio affiliate near Lake Norman in North Carolina where she lives.

In 1997 Myelita started SpeakEasy Communications to offer industry specific Spanish instruction in the Carolinas. The company is now the nation's leader in Spanish training, offering over 30 *SpeakEasy Spanish*™ programs and publications to companies, associations, and colleges throughout the US.

Lita is also a member of the National Speaker's Association and the National Council for Continuing Education and Training. Many of her clients say she is the most high-energy, results-oriented speaker they have ever seen. As she travels the country speaking on cultural diversity issues in the workplace and languages, she is realizing her dream of being able to s to the world.

English Spanish Dictionary

A

A little = Un poco
A lot = Mucho
A or an = Un *(m)*, Una *(f)*
Abdomen = Abdomen
Abnormal = Anormal
Above = Encima
Abscess = Absceso
Address = Dirección
Afraid of = Miedo de
After meals = Después de las comidas
Age = Edad
AIDS = SIDA, Síndrome de inmunodeficiencia adquirida
Aisle = Pasillo
Allergies = Alergias
Ampule = Ampolleta
Analgesic = Analgésico
Anemia = Anemia
Anesthetic = Anestésico
Ankle = Tobillo
Answering machine = Contestador telefónico
Antacid = Antiácido
Antibiotic = Antibiótico
Anticoagulant = Anticoagulante
Antidote = Antídoto
Antihistamine = Antihistamínicos
Anti-inflammatory = Anti-inflamatorio
Antiseptic = Antiséptico
Anus = Ano
Anxiety = Ansiedad
Apartment number = Número de apartamento
Appendicitis = Apendicitis
Apply = Aplique
April = abril
Are you sure = Está seguro (a)
Are you using herbal products = Usa productos naturales o remedios caseros
Are you using home remedies = Usa remedios caseros
Are you using over the counter medications = Usa medicinas sin receta médica
Area code = Código de área
Arm = Brazo
Around = Alrededor
Arrhythmias = Palpitaciones
Arthritis = Artritis

As directed by your doctor = Según las instrucciones de su doctor.
Ashamed = Vergüenza
Ask for this number. = Pida este número.
Aspirin = Aspirina
Assistant = Ayudante
Asthma = Asma
Astringent = Astringente
At bedtime = A la hora de acostarse
August = agosto
Aunt = Tía
Avenue = Avenida

B

Back = Espalda
Backache = Dolor de espalda
Bacteria = Bacteria
Bacterial infection = Infección bacteriana
Bad = Mal
Bad reaction = Mala reacción
Barbiturate = Barbitúrico
Basement = Sótano
Before meals = Antes de las comidas
Behind = Detrás
Beside = Al lado de
Between meals = Entre las comidas
Big = Grande
Black = Negro
Bladder infection = Infección de vejiga
Bleeding = Sangrado
Blister = Ampolla
Blood = Sangre
Blood pressure = Presión arterial Presión sanguínea, Tensión arterial
Blood sugar = Glucosa en la sangre
Blue = Azul
Blurred vision = Visión borrosa
Body = Cuerpo
Boss = Jefe , *(m)* Jefa *(f)*
Bottle = Botella
Brain = Cerebro
Bring me that = Tráigame eso.
Broken bone = Hueso roto
Bronchitis = Bronquitis
Brother = Hermano
Brother-in-law = Cuñado
Brown = Moreno

Bruise = Contusión
Bump = Hinchazón
Burn = Quemadura
By mouth = Por boca

C

Cafeteria = Cafetería
Calm down = Cálmese
Cancer = Cáncer
Canine = Diente canino
Capsule = Cápsula
Carbohydrates = Carbohidratos
Carry this. = Lleve esto
Cellular phone = Teléfono celular
Cheek = Mejilla
Chemotherapy = Quimioterapia
Chest = Pecho
Chest pain = Dolor de pecho
Chicken pox = Varicela
Child = Niño *(m)*, Niña *(f)*
Chills = Escalofrío
Chin = Barbilla
Chronic fatigue = Cansancio crónico
Close = Cierra
Codeine = Codeína
Cold (chest) = Gripe
Cold *(ill)* = Catarro
Cold *(phy)* = Frío
Colic = Cólico
Collect call = Llamada a cobro revertido
Come back soon. = Regrese pronto.
Come here = Venga aquí
Condition = Condición
Condom = Condón
Conference call = Llamada de conferencia
Constipation = Estreñimiento
Contact = Contacto
Contraceptive = Contraceptivo
Cortisone = Cortisona
Cough = Tos
Cough drop = Pastillas para la tos
Cough syrup = Jarabe para la tos
Could you call later = Puede llamar más tarde
Cousin = Primo *(m)*, Prima *(f)*
Cramps = Calambres
Cream = Crema
Cup = Una copa
Cyst = Quiste

D

Dark = Oscuro
Date of birth = Fecha de nacimiento
Daughter = Hija
Daughter-in-law = Nuera
December = diciembre
Decrease of appetite = Disminución del apetito
Department = Departamento
Depression = Depresión
Diabetes = Diabetes
Diabetic = Diabético (a)
Dial this number. = Marque este número.
Diaper rash = Exantema del pañal
Diarrhea = Diarrea
Disinfectant = Desinfectante
Diuretic = Diurético
Divorced = Divorciado (a)
Dizziness = Mareos, Vértigo
Do it later. = Hágalo más tarde
Do it now = Hágalo ahora
Do you have a lot of pain = Tiene mucho dolor
Do you have insurance for your medication = Tiene seguro para su medicina
Do you have pain = Tiene dolor
Do you need a refill = Necesita un relleno
Do you speak English = Habla inglés
Do you understand = Comprende
Doctor = Doctor, *(m)* Doctora *(f)*
Does it hurt = Le duele
Don't swallow = No traiga
Don't worry = No se preocupe
Dosage = Dosis
Down = Abajo
Driver's license number = Número de licencia
Drop = Gota
Dropper = Cuentagotas
Dry mouth = Boca seca

E

Ear = Oreja
Ear canal = Conducto auditivo, Canal
Ear drops = Gotas para el oído
Ear drum = Tímpano
Earache = Dolor de oído
East = Este

Eczema = Eccema
Eight = Ocho
Eight hundred = Ochocientos
Eight hundred number = Número de ochocientos
Eighteen = Diez y ocho
Eighty = Ochenta
Elevator = Ascensor
Eleven = Once
Emergency room = Sala de emergencia
Energy = Energía
Entrance = Entrada
Erectile dysfunction = Disfunción eréctil
Every ____ hours = Cada ____ horas
Every day = Cada día
Excellent = Excelente
Excessive = Excesivo (a)
Excuse me = Perdón
Exercise = Ejercicio
Exit = Salida
Expiration date = Fecha de expiración
Extension = Extensión
Externally = Externamente
Eye = Ojo
Eye drops = Gotas para los ojos
Eyebrow = Ceja
Eyelash = Pestaña
Eyelid = Párpado

F

Face = Cara
Fantastic = Fantástico
Far = Lejos
Fast acting = Acción rápida
Father = Padre
Father-in-law = Suegro
Fax = Facsímile
February = febrero
Fever = Fiebre
Fifteen = Quince
Fifty = Cincuenta
Fine = Muy bien.
Finger = Dedo
First name = Primer nombre
Five = Cinco
Five hundred = Quinientos
Flu = Influenza
Fluid retention = Retención de flujo
Fluids = Fluidos
Foot = Pie
For # months = Por # meses
For # weeks = Por # semanas

For # days = Por # días
For external use = Para uso externo
Forehead = Frente
Forty = Cuarenta
Four = Cuatro
Four hundred = Cuatrocientos
Fourteen = Catorce
Frequent urination = Orina con frecuencia
Friday = viernes
Fruit juice = Jugo de frutas
Full name = Nombre completo
Fungus = Hongo

G

Gall stones = Cálculos en la vesícula
Gargle = Hace gárgaras
Gift shop = Tienda de regalos
Give it to me = Démelo.
Glass = Un vaso
Glaucoma = Glaucoma
Glucometer = Glucómetro
Glucose = Glucosa
Go with him = Vaya con él
Gold = Oro
Good afternoon = Buenas tardes
Good idea. = Buena idea.
Good luck = Buena suerte
Good morning = Buenos días
Good night = Buenas noches.
Good-bye = Adiós
Gout = Gota
Granddaughter = Nieta
Grandfather = Abuelo
Grandmother = Abuela
Grandson = Nieto
Gray = Gris
Green = Verde
Gums = Encías

H

Half = Una media
Hall = Corredor
Hand = Mano
Hang up the telephone. = Cuelgue el teléfono.
Happy birthday = Feliz cumpleaños
Hard palate = Paladar duro

Have a nice day = Qué le vaya bien, Tenga un buen día.

Hay fever = Fiebre de heno

He = Él

He/She isn't here. = No está aquí.

He/she will call back later. = Llamará más tarde.

He's precious
She's precious = Es precioso, Es preciosa

Head = Cabeza

Head ache = Dolor de cabeza

Headset = Auriculares con micrófono

Heart = Corazón

Help him = Ayúdelo

Help me = Ayúdeme

Hemoglobin = Hemoglobina

Hepatitis = Hepatitis

Here = Aquí

Herpes = Herpes

Hi = Hola

Hiccups = Hipo

High = Alto (a)

High blood pressure = Presión arterial alta, Presión alta

His, her or Your (polite) = Su, Sus

HIV = VIH, Virus de la inmunodeficiencia humana

Hives = Urticaria, Ronchas de la piel

Hold a moment = Espere un momento

Home telephone number = Número de teléfono de su casa

Hot = Caliente

Housekeeper = Doméstico (a)

How = Cómo

How are you = Cómo está

How do you say it in Spanish = Cómo se dice en español

How many = Cuántos

How much = Cuánto

How old is your baby = Cuántos años tiene su bebé

How pretty = Qué bonito (m), Qué bonita (f), Qué lindo (m), Qué linda (f)

Hungry = Hambre

Husband = Esposo

Hyperglycemia = Hiperglicemia

Hypertension = Hipotensión

Hyperthyroidism = Hipertiroidismo

Hypoglycemia = Hipoglucemia

I

I = Yo

I agree. = De acuerdo.

I am going to call your doctor for authorization to renew this prescription. = Voy a llamar a su doctor para que autorice la repetición de esta receta médica.

I am going to call your doctor. = Voy a llamar a su doctor.

I believe so. = Creo que sí.

I don't understand. = No comprendo.

I have the wrong number. = Tengo el número equivocado.

I need your insurance card, please. = Necesito su tarjeta de seguro, por favor.

I speak a little Spanish. = Hablo poco español.

I'd like to leave a message. = Me gustaría dejar un mensaje.

I'll transfer you to = Le voy a transferir a _____

I'm calling about = Estoy llamando acerca de

I'm going to look for a translator = Voy a buscar un traductor

I'm so glad = Me alegro

I'm sorry = Lo siento

I'm studying Spanish = Estudio español

I'll be right back = Ahora vengo

I'm leaving now = Ya me voy

I'm sorry. = Lo siento.

Immune system = Sistema inmunitario

In front of = En frente de

In pain. = Dolor

In the afternoon = Por la tarde

In the evening = Por la noche

In the morning = Por la mañana

Incisor = Diente incisivo

Increase of appetite = Aumento del apetito

Indigestion = Indigestión

Infection = Infección

Inflammation = Inflamación

Inhale = Inhale

Inhaler = Inhalador

Injection = Inyección

Inner ear = Oído

In-patient = Paciente interno

Insert = Inserta

Inside = Adentro

Insomnia = Insomnio

Insulin = Insulina

Intensive care = Cuidados intensivos
Intermediate acting = Acción intermedia
Is the pain burning = Tiene dolor quemante
Is the pain constant = Tiene dolor constante
Is the pain deep = Tiene dolor profundo
Is the pain intermittent = Tiene dolor intermitente
Is the pain mild = Tiene dolor moderado
Is the pain severe = Tiene dolor muy fuerte
Is the pain throbbing = Tiene dolor pulsante
Is this the correct number = Es el número correcto
It hurts. = Me duele.
It will take # minutes to prepare. = Necesito # minutos prepararla.
It's important. = Es importante.
It's serious. = Es grave.
It's very important. = Es muy importante.
Itching = Picazón
It's possible. = Es posible

J
Janitor = Portero *(a)*
January = enero
Jaundice = Ictericia
July = julio
June = junio

K
Keep refrigerated = Guarda en el refrigerador
Ketoacidosis = Quetoacidosis
Ketone = Quejona
Kidney stones = Cálculos en los riñones
Knee = Rodilla
Knee = Rodilla

L
Label = Etiqueta
Laboratory = Laboratorio
Lancet = Lanceta
Laryngitis = Laringitis
Last name (*surname*) = Apellido

Laxative = Laxante
Leg = Pierna
Less = Menos
Let's go = Vámonos
Leukemia = Leucemia
Level = Nivel
Lice = Piojos
Ligament = Ligamento
Light = Claro
Like this = Así
Liniment = Linimento
Little = Pequeño
Lobby = Salón
Local call = Llamada local
Long distance = Larga distancia
Long lasting = Dura mucho tiempo
Lotion = Loción
Low = Bajo *(a)*
Low blood pressure = Presión arterial baja
Lozenge = Pastilla
Lump = Bulto

M
March = marzo
Marital status = Estado civil
Married = Casado *(a)*
Maternal surname = Apellido materno
Maternity = Maternidad
May = mayo
May I help you = Puedo servirle
May I speak to = Puedo hablar con
Maybe. = Quizás.
Me neither = Yo tampoco
Me too = Yo también
Measles = Sarampión
Menstrual pain = Dolor de la menstruación
Middle name = Segundo nombre
Migraine = Jaqueca, Migraña
Milliliter = Mililitro
Miss = Señorita
Mix = Mezclar
Molar = Muela , Molar
Monday = lunes
Monitor = Monitor
Mononucleosis = Mononucleosis
More = Más
Morphine = Morfina
Mother = Madre
Mother-in-law = Suegra

Motion sickness = Mareo
Mouth = Boca
Move that here = Mueve eso aquí
Mrs. or Ma'am = Señora
Mumps = Paperas
My = Mi, Mis
My name is = Me llamo

N

Nail = Uña
Narcotic = Narcótico
Nasal decongestant = Descongestionante nasal
Nationality = Nacionalidad
Nausea = Náusea
Near = Cerca de
Neck = Cuello
Needle = Aguja
Nephew = Sobrino
Nice to meet you. = Mucho gusto
Niece = Sobrina
Nine = Nueve
Nineteen = Diez y nueve
Ninety = Noventa
Ninety = Novecientos
Nitroglycerine = Nitroglicerina
No refills = No hay rellenos, No hay repeticiones, No se puede repetir
Normal = Normal
North = Norte
Nose = Nariz
Not like this = Así no
November = noviembre
NPH insulin = Insulina NPH
Number = Español
Numbness or tingling in the hands or feet = Adormecimiento u hormigueo en las manos o pies
Nurse = Enfermera (o)
Nutritional Supplement = Suplemento nutricional

O

Occupation = Ocupación
October = octubre
On an empty stomach = Con el estómago vacío.
One = Uno
One drop = Una gota

One half teaspoon = Una media cucharadita
One hundred = Cien
One moment please = Un momento, por favor
One quarter = Un cuarto
One tablespoon = Una cucharada
One teaspoon = Una cucharadita
One third = Un tercero
One thousand = Mil
Only when necessary = Solo cuando es necesario
Only when you have pain = Solo cuando tiene dolor
Open = Abre
Operating room = Sala de operaciones
Oral sex = Sexo oral
Orange = Naranja
Oropharynx = Orofaringe
Our = Nuestro *(-os)*, Nuestra *(-as)*
Outer ear = Oreja
Out-patient = Paciente externo
Outside = Afuera
Over there = Allá
Overweight = Sobrepeso

P

Pain = Dolor
Pancreas = Páncreas
Paramedic = Paramédico
Parking lot = Estacionamiento
Patch = Parche
Paternal surname = Apellido paterno
Patient = Paciente
Pediatrics = Pediátrico
Penicillin = Penicilina
Penis = Pene
Pharmacist = Farmacéutico *(a)*
Photosensitivity = Sensibilidad a la luz solar
Physical therapy = Terapia física
Pick up all these = Recoja todo esto
Pill = Píldora
Pink = Rosa
Place of birth = Lugar de nacimiento
Place of employment = Lugar de empleo
Please = Por favor
Please contact your doctor = Favor de consultar a su doctor.
Please hold a moment = Favor de esperar un momento.

Please sign here = Favor de firmar aquí
Please sit over there = Favor de sentarse allá
Please wait = Favor de esperar
PMS = Síndrome premenstrual
Pneumonia = Pulmonía, Neumonía
Point to it = Indícalo.
Police = Policía
Pregnant = Embarazada
Premixed insulin = Insulina premezclada
Prescription = Receta médica, Fórmula, Receta
Press this number = Oprima este número
Protection = Protección
Psoriasis = Psoriasis
Pupil = Pupila
Purple = Morado
Put it there = Póngalo allí

Q
Quantity = Cantidad

R
Radiology = Radiología
Rain = Lluvia
Rash = Erupción
Really = De veras
Receptionist = Recepcionista
Recovery room = Sala de recuperación
Rectal Suppository = Supositorio rectal
Rectum = Recto
Red = Rojo
Refrigerator = Refrigerador
Regular insulin = Insulina regular
Remove these = Quite estos
Repeat, please. = Repita, por favor.
Resistance = Resistencia
Respiratory therapy = Terapia respiratoria
Rest rooms = Sanitarios, Baño
Right = Razón
Risk = Riesgo

S
Safety cap = Tapón de seguridad
Saline = Salina
Saturday = sábado
Secretary = Secretaria

Security guard = Guardia de seguridad
Sedative = Sedante
Semen = Semen
Separated = Separado (a)
September = septiembre
Seven = Siete
Seven hundred = Setecientos
Seventeen = Diez y siete
Seventy = Setenta
Sex = Sexo
Sexual problems = Problemas sexuales
Sexual relations = Coito sexual
Shake well = Agítese bien
She = Ella
Shortness of breath = Respiración corta
Shoulder = Hombro
Show me. = Indícalo.
Sick = Enfermo
Silver = Plata
Single = Soltero *(a)*
Sir or Mister = Señor
Sister = Hermana
Sister-in-law = Cuñada
Six = Seis
Six hundred = Seiscientos
Sixteen = Diez y seis
Sixty = Sesenta
Skin = Piel
Skin = Piel
Sleep = Dormir
Sleepiness = Sueño
Sleepy = Sueño
Snack = Merienda
So so = Así así
Social security number = Número de seguro social
Soft palate = Paladar blando
Solution = Solución
Some *(pl)* = Unos, Unas
Son = Hijo
Son-in-law = Yerno
Sore throat = Dolor de garganta
South = Sur
Sparingly = Poco
Speak more slowly = Habla más despacio
Spine = Espina
Spit = Escupe
Sprain = Torcedura
Spray = Rociada
Stairs = Escaleras
Step daughter = Hijastra
Step father = Padrastro

Step mother = Madrastra
Step son = Hijastro
Steroid = Esteroide
Stomach = Estómago
Stomach pain = Dolor de estómago
Stop = Pare
Straight ahead = Adelante
Street = Calle
Stress = Estrés
Stuffy nose = Nariz tupida
Stye = Orzuelo
Sudden weight loss = Pérdida súbita de peso
Sugar = Azúcar
Sunday = domingo
Supervisor = Supervisor , Supervisora
Suppositories = Supositorios
Sure = Claro
Swallow = Traiga
Sweats = Sudores
Swelling = Inflamación, Hinchazón
Swish = Susurro
Switchboard = Conmutador
Symptoms = Síntomas
Syringe = Jeringuilla

T

Tablet = Tableta, Pastilla
Take = Toma
Take _____ times = Toma _____ veces
Take the medicine = Toma la medicina
Take the medicine # times per day = Toma la medicina # veces por día
Tear duct = Conducto lagrimar
Teeth = Dientes
Telephone = Teléfono
Telephone number = Número de teléfono
Ten = Diez
Tendon = Tendón
Thank you for waiting = Gracias para esperando
Thank you = Gracias
Thanks for your patience = Gracias por su paciencia
That depends = Depende
That's OK = Está bien
The = El (m), La (f), Los (mpl), Las (fpl)
The connection is bad = La conexión está mala
The line is busy = La línea está ocupada

The number is disconnected = El número está desconectado
The pleasure is mine = El gusto es mío
Therapist = Terapeuta
Therapy = Terapia
There = Allí
There = Allí
There is a phone call for = Hay una llamada para
They = Ellos (mpl), Ellas (fpl)
They hurt = Me duelen
Thighs = Muslos
Thirsty = Sed
Thirteen = Trece
Thirty = Treinta
Three = Tres
Three hundred = Trescientos
Throat = Garganta
Throat = Garganta
Thursday = jueves
Times per day = veces al día
To affected areas = En las áreas afectadas
To ask = Preguntar
To be cold = Hace frío
To be cool = Hace fresco
To be hot = Hace calor
To be nice weather = Hace buen tiempo
To be sunny = Hace sol
To be windy = Hace viento
To call = Llamar
To control = Controlar
To cooperate = Cooperar
To fill = Llenar
To forget = Olvidar
To listen to = Escuchar
To look at = Mirar
To measure = Medir
To need = Necesitar
To observe = Observar
To pay = Pagar
To prepare = Preparar
To prevent = Prevenir
To rain. = Llover
To return = Regresar
To take = Tomar
To the left = A la izquierda
To the right = A la derecha
To use = Usar
To verify = Verificar
To work = Trabajar
Toe = Dedo del pie
Tongue = Lengua

Tonsil = Amígdala
Tooth = Diente
Tooth = Diente
Tooth ache = Dolor del diente
Tranquilizers = Tranquilizantes
Transmission = Transmisión
Tremor = Temblor
Tuberculosis = Tuberculosis
Tuesday = martes
Turn = Doble
Twelve = Doce
Twenty = Veinte
Twenty eight = Veinte y ocho
Twenty five = Veinte y cinco
Twenty four = Veinte y cuatro
Twenty nine = Veinte y nueve
Twenty one = Veinte y uno
Twenty seven = Veinte y siete
Twenty six = Veinte y seis
Twenty three = Veinte y tres
Twenty two = Veinte y dos
Two = Dos
Two hundred = Doscientos
Two-way radio = Radioteléfono portátil
Type 1 = Tipo uno
Type 2 = Tipo dos

U

Ulcer = Úlcera
Uncle = Tío
Under = Debajo
Until finished = Hasta que se termina
Unwrap = Desempaqueta
Up = Arriba
Urine = Orina
Use for = Use para
Using the numbers from one through ten indicate the level of your pain. = Usando los números de uno hasta diez, indique el nivel de su dolor.
Uvula = Úvula

V

Vaccine = Vacuna
Vagina = Vagina
Vaginal infections = Infecciones vaginales
Vaginal Suppository = Supositorio vaginal
Vapor nebulizer = Nebulizador de vapor

Vial = Vial
Virus = Virus
Visitor = Visitante
Vitamins = Vitaminas
Vomiting = Vomitando

W

Wait = Espere
Wait for the tone. = Espere por el tono.
Waiting room = Sala de espera
Water fountain = Fuente de agua
We = Nosotros, Nosotras (f)
We appreciate your business. = Apreciamos su negocio.
We'll see you. = Nos vemos.
Weakness = Debilidad
Wednesday = miércoles
Weight gain = Aumento de peso
West = Oeste
What = Qué
What a smile = Qué sonrisa
What is your doctor's name = Cuál es el nombre de su doctor
What is your doctor's telephone number = Cuál es el número de teléfono de su doctor
What time is it = Qué hora es
What's happening = Qué pasa
What's the weather = Qué tiempo hace
What's your baby's name = Cómo se llama su bebé
What's your name = Cómo se llama
When = Cuándo
Where = Dónde
Where = Dónde
Where are you from = De dónde es
Which = Cuál
White = Blanco
Who = Quién
Why = Por qué
Widow = Viudo (a)
Wife = Esposa
With breakfast = Con el desayuno
With dinner = Con la cena
With food = Con la comida
With lunch = Con el almuerzo
With milk = Con leche
With water = Con agua
Without protection = Sin protección
Work telephone number = Número de teléfono de su empleo

Would you like to leave a message = Le gustaría
dejar un mensaje
Would you like to wait for your
prescription = Le gusta esperar para
su receta médica
Wound = Herida
Wounds that won't heal = Heridas que
no sanan
Wrist = Muñeca
Write it, please = Escribe, por favor.
X-ray = Rayos equis
xx years old = xx años

Y

Yeast infection = Infección de levadura
Yellow = Amarillo
You (informal) = Tú
You (Polite) = Usted
You have the wrong number. = Tiene el
número equivocado.
You may repeat this once. = Se puede
repetir esta una vez.
You may repeat this prescription #
times. = Se puede repetir esta receta
médica # veces.
You're welcome = De nada
Your = Tu, Tus *(pl)*
Your doctor changed your prescription.
= Su doctor se cambió su receta
médica.
Your name, please = Su nombre, por
favor
Your number, please = Su número, por
favor
Your prescription will be ready this
afternoon. = Su receta médica estará
lista esta tarde.
Your prescription will be ready
tomorrow. = Su receta médica estará
lista mañana.
Your total is # dollars. = Su cuenta está
dólares.

Z

Zero = Cero

Spanish-English Dictionary

A

A la derecha = To the right
A la hora de acostarse = At bedtime
A la izquierda = To the left
Abajo = Down
Abdomen = Abdomen
Abre = Open
abril = April
Absceso = Abscess
Abuela = Grandmother
Abuelo = Grandfather
Acción intermedia = Intermediate acting
Acción rápida = Fast acting
Adelante = Straight ahead
Adentro = Inside
Adiós = Good-bye
Adormecimiento u hormigueo en las
manos o pies = Numbness or tingling in
the hands or feet
Afuera = Outside
Agítese bien = Shake well
agosto = August
Agujas = Needles
Ahora vengo = I'll be right back
Al lado de = Beside
Alergias = Allergies
Allá = Over there
Allí = There
Alrededor = Around
Alto *(a)* = High
Amarillo = Yellow
Amígdala = Tonsil
Ampolla = Blister
Ampolleta = Ampule
Analgésico = Analgesic
Anemia = Anemia
Anestésico = Anesthetic
Ano = Anus
Anormal = Abnormal
Ansiedad = Anxiety
Antes de las comidas = Before meals
Antiácido = Antacid
Antibiótico = Antibiotic
Anticoagulante = Anticoagulant
Antídoto = Antidote
Antihistamínicos = Antihistamine
Anti-inflamatorio = Anti-inflammatory
Antiséptico = Antiseptic

Apellido = Last name *(surname)*
Apellido materno = Maternal surname
Apellido paterno = Paternal surname
Apendicitis = Appendicitis
Aplique = Apply
Apreciamos su negocio = We appreciate your business
Aquí = Here
Arriba = Up
Artritis = Arthritis
Ascensor = Elevator
Así = Like this
Así así = So so
Así no = Not like this
Asma = Asthma
Aspirina = Aspirin
Astringente = Astringent
Aumento de peso = Weight gain
Aumento del apetito = Increase of appetite
Auriculares con micrófono = Headset
Avenida = Avenue
Ayudante = Assistant
Ayúdelo = Help him
Ayúdeme = Help me
Azúcar = Sugar
Azul = Blue

B

Bacteria = Bacteria
Bajo *(a)* = Low
Barbilla = Chin
Barbitúrico = Barbiturate
Blanco = White
Boca = Mouth
Boca seca = Dry mouth
Botella = Bottle
Brazo = Arm
Bronquitis = Bronchitis
Buena idea. = Good idea.
Buena suerte = Good luck
Buenas noches. = Good night
Buenas tardes = Good afternoon
Buenos días = Good morning
Bulto = Lump

C

Cabeza = Head
Cada # horas = Every # hours
Cada día = Every day

Cafetería = Cafeteria
Calambres = Cramps
Cálculos en la vesícula = Gall stones
Cálculos en los riñones = Kidney stones
Caliente = Hot
Calle = Street
Cálmese = Calm down
Cáncer = Cancer
Cansancio crónico = Chronic fatigue
Cantidad = Quantity
Cápsula = Capsule
Cara = Face
Carbohidratos = Carbohydrates
Casado *(a)* = Married
Catarro = Cold *(ill)*
Catorce = Fourteen
Ceja = Eyebrow
Cerca de = Near
Cerebro = Brain
Cero = Zero
Cien = One hundred
Cierra = Close
Cinco = Five
Cincuenta = Fifty
Claro = Light
Claro = Sure
Codeína = Codeine
Código de área = Area code
Coito sexual = Sexual relations
Cólico = Colic
Cómo = How
Cómo está = How are you
Cómo se dice en español = How do you say it in Spanish
Cómo se llama = What's your name
Cómo se llama su bebé = What's your baby's name
Comprende = Do you understand
Con agua = With water
Con el almuerzo = With lunch
Con el desayuno = With breakfast
Con el estómago vacío = On an empty stomach
Con la cena = With dinner
Con la comida = With food
Con leche = With milk
Condición = Condition
Condón = Condom
Conducto auditivo, Canal = Ear canal
Conducto lagrimar = Tear duct
Conmutador = Switchboard
Contacto = Contact

Contestador telefónico = Answering machine
Contraceptivo = Contraceptive
Controlar = To control
Contusión = Bruise
Cooperar = To cooperate
Copa = Cup
Corazón = Heart
Corredor = Hall
Cortisona = Cortisone
Crema = Cream
Creo que sí. = I believe so.
Cuál = Which, What
Cuál es el nombre de su doctor = What is your doctor's name
Cuál es el número de teléfono de su doctor = What is your doctor's telephone number
Cuándo = When
Cuánto = How much
Cuántos = How many
Cuántos años tiene su bebé = How old is your baby
Cuarenta = Forty
Cuatro = Four
Cuatrocientos = Four hundred
Cucharada = One tablespoon
Cucharadita = One teaspoon
Cuelgue el teléfono = Hang up the telephone
Cuello = Neck
Cuentagotas = Dropper
Cuerpo = Body
Cuidados intensivos = Intensive care
Cuñada = Sister-in-law
Cuñado = Brother-in-law

D

De acuerdo = I agree
De dónde es = Where are you from
De nada = You're welcome
De veras = Really
Debajo = Under
Debilidad = Weakness
Dedo = Finger
Dedo del pie = Toe
Démelo = Give it to me
Dentro = Inside
Departamento = Department
Depende = That depends
Depresión = Depression

Descongestionante nasal = Nasal decongestant
Desempaqueta = Unwrap
Desinfectante = Disinfectant
Después de las comidas = After meals
Detrás = Behind
Diabetes = Diabetes
Diabético (a) = Diabetic
Diarrea = Diarrhea
diciembre = December
Diente = Tooth
Diente = Tooth
Diente canino = Canine
Diente incisivo = Incisor
Dientes = Teeth
Diez = Ten
Diez y nueve = Nineteen
Diez y ocho = Eighteen
Diez y seis = Sixteen
Diez y siete = Seventeen
Dirección = Address
Disfunción eréctil = Erectile dysfunction
Disminución del apetito = Decrease of appetite
Diurético = Diuretic
Divorciado (a) = Divorced
Doble = Turn
Doce = Twelve
Doctor, (m) Doctora (f) = Doctor
Dolor = Pain
Dolor de cabeza = Head ache
Dolor de espalda = Backache
Dolor de estómago = Stomach pain
Dolor de garganta = Sore throat
Dolor de la menstruación = Menstrual pain
Dolor de oído = Earache
Dolor de pecho = Chest pain
Dolor del diente = Tooth ache
Doméstico (a) = Housekeeper
domingo = Sunday
Dónde = Where
Dormir = Sleep
Dos = Two
Doscientos = Two hundred
Dosis = Dosage
Dura mucho tiempo = Long lasting

E

Eccema = Eczema
Edad = Age
Ejercicio = Exercise

Él = He
El *(m)*, La *(f),* Los *(mpl)*, Las *(fpl)* = The
El gusto es mío = The pleasure is mine
El número está desconectado = The number is disconnected
Ella = She
Ellos *(mpl)*, Ellas *(fpl)* = They
Embarazada = Pregnant
En frente de = In front of
En las áreas afectadas = To affected areas
Encías = Gums
Encima = Above
Energía = Energy
enero = January
Enfermera (o) = Nurse
Enfermo = Sick
Entrada = Entrance
Entre las comidas = Between meals
Erupción = Rash
Erupción = Rash
Erupción = Rash
Es el número correcto = Is this the correct number
Es grave = It's serious
Es importante = It's important
Es muy importante = It's very important
Es posible = It's possible
Es precioso, Es preciosa = He's precious, She's precious
Escaleras = Stairs
Escalofrío = Chills
Escribe = Write it
Escuchar = To listen to
Escupe = Spit
Espalda = Back
Español = Number
Espere = Wait
Espere por el tono. = Wait for the tone.
Espere un momento = Hold a moment,
Espina = Spine
Esposa = Wife
Esposo = Husband
Está bien = That's OK
Está seguro *(a)* = Are you sure
Estacionamiento = Parking lot
Estado civil = Marital status
Este = East
Esteroide = Steroid
Estómago = Stomach
Estoy llamando acerca de = I'm calling about
Estreñimiento = Constipation

Estrés = Stress
Estudio español = I'm studying Spanish.
Etiqueta = Label
Exantema del pañal = Diaper rash
Excelente = Excellent
Excesivo (a) = Excessive
Extensión = Extension
Externamente = Externally

F
Facsímile = Fax
Fantástico = Fantastic
Farmacéutico *(a)* = Pharmacist
Favor de consultar a su doctor. = Please contact your doctor
Favor de esperar = Please wait
Favor de esperar un momento = Please hold a moment
Favor de firmar aquí = Please sign here
Favor de sentarse allá = Please sit over there
febrero = February
Fecha de expiración = Expiration date
Fecha de nacimiento = Date of birth
Feliz cumpleaños = Happy birthday
Fiebre = Fever
Fiebre de heno = Hay fever
Fluidos = Fluids
Frente = Forehead
Frío = Cold *(phy)*
Fuente de agua = Water fountain

G
Garganta = Throat
Garganta = Throat
Glaucoma = Glaucoma
Glucómetro = Glucometer
Glucosa = Glucose
Glucosa en la sangre = Blood sugar
Gota = Drop
Gota = Drop
Gotas para el oído = Ear drops
Gotas para los ojos = Eye drops
Gracias = Thank you
Gracias para esperando = Thank you for waiting
Gracias por su paciencia = Thanks for your patience
Grande = Big
Gripe = Cold (*chest*)
Gris = Gray

124

Guarda en el refrigerador = Keep refrigerated
Guardia de seguridad = Security guard

H
Habla inglés = Do you speak English
Habla más despacio = Speak more slowly
Hablo poco español = I speak a little Spanish
Hace buen tiempo = To be nice weather
Hace calor = To be hot
Hace fresco = To be cool
Hace frío = To be cold
Hace gárgaras = Gargle
Hace sol = To be sunny
Hace viento = To be windy
Hágalo ahora = Do it now
Hágalo más tarde = Do it later
Hambre = Hungry
Hasta que se termina = Until finished
Hay una llamada para = There is a phone call for
Hemoglobina = Hemoglobin
Hepatitis = Hepatitis
Herida = Wound
Heridas que no sanan = Wounds that won't heal
Hermana = Sister
Hermano = Brother
Herpes = Herpes
Hija = Daughter
Hijastra = Step daughter
Hijastro = Step son
Hijo = Son
Hinchazón = Bump
Hiperglicemia = Hyperglycemia
Hipertiroidismo = Hyperthyroidism
Hipo = Hiccups
Hipoglucemia = Hypoglycemia
Hipotensión = Hypertension
Hola = Hi
Hombro = Shoulder
Hongo = Fungus
Hueso roto = Broken bone

I
Indícalo = Show me.
Indícalo. = Point to it
Indigestión = Indigestion
Infección = Infection

Infección bacteriana = Bacterial infection
Infección de levadura = Yeast infection
Infección de vejiga = Bladder infection
Infeccion vaginal = Vaginal infection
Inflamación = Inflammation
Inflamación = Swelling
Influenza = Flu
Inhalador = Inhaler
Inhale = Inhale
Inserta = Insert
Insomnio = Insomnia
Insulina = Insulin
Insulina NPH = NPH insulin
Insulina premezclada = Premixed insulin
Insulina regular = Regular insulin
Inyección = Injection

J
Jaqueca, Migraña = Migraine
Jarabe para la tos = Cough syrup
Jefe , *(m)* Jefa *(f)* = Boss
Jeringuilla = Syringe
jueves = Thursday
Jugo de frutas = Fruit juice
julio = July
junio = June

L
La conexión está mala = The connection is bad
La línea está ocupada = The line is busy
Laboratorio = Laboratory
Lanceta = Lancet
Larga distancia = Long distance
Laringitis = Laryngitis
Laxante = Laxative
Le duele = Does it hurt
Le gusta esperar para su receta médica = Would you like to wait for your prescription
Le gustaría dejar un mensaje = Would you like to leave a message
Le voy a transferir a = I'll transfer you to
Lejos = Far
Lengua = Tongue
Leucemia = Leukemia
Ligamento = Ligament
Linimento = Liniment

Llamada a cobro revertido = Collect call
Llamada de conferencia = Conference call
Llamada local = Local call
Llamar = To call
Llamará más tarde. = He/she will call back later.
Llenar = To fill
Lleve esto = Carry this.
Llover = To rain.
Lluvia = Rain
Lo siento = I'm sorry.
Loción = Lotion
Lugar de empleo = Place of employment
Lugar de nacimiento = Place of birth
lunes = Monday

M

Madrastra = Step mother
Madre = Mother
Mal = Bad
Mala reacción = Bad reaction
Mano = Hand
Mareo = Motion sickness
Mareos, Vértigo = Dizziness
Marque este número. = Dial this number.
martes = Tuesday
marzo = March
Más = More
Maternidad = Maternity
mayo = May
Me alegro = I'm so glad
Me duele = It hurts
Me duelen = They hurt
Me gustaría dejar un mensaje = I'd like to leave a message
Me llamo = My name is
Media cucharadita = One half teaspoon
Medir = To measure
Mejilla = Cheek
Menos = Less
Merienda = Snack
Mezclar = Mix
Mi, Mis = My
Miedo de = Afraid of
miércoles = Wednesday
Mil = One thousand
Mililitro = Milliliter
Mirar = To look at
Monitor = Monitor
Mononucleosis = Mononucleosis

Morado = Purple
Moreno = Brown
Morfina = Morphine
Mucho = A lot
Mucho gusto = Nice to meet you
Muela, Molar = Molar
Mueve eso aquí = Move that here
Muñeca = Wrist
Muñeca = Wrist
Muslos = Thighs
Muy bien. = Fine

N

Nacionalidad = Nationality
Naranja = Orange
Narcótico = Narcotic
Nariz = Nose
Nariz tupida = Stuffy nose
Náusea = Nausea
Nebulizador de vapor = Vapor nebulizer
Necesita un relleno = Do you need a refill
Necesitar = To need
Necesito # minutos prepararla = It will take # minutes to prepare
Necesito su tarjeta de seguro = I need your insurance card
Negro = Black
Nieta = Granddaughter
Nieto = Grandson
Niño (m), Niña (f) = Child
Nitroglicerina = Nitroglycerine
Nivel = Level
No comprendo = I don't understand
No está aquí = He/She isn't here
No hay rellenos, No hay repeticiones, No se puede repetir = No refills
No se preocupe = Don't worry
No traiga = Don't swallow
Nombre completo = Full name
Normal = Normal
Norte = North
Nos vemos. = We'll see you.
Nos vemos. = We'll see you.
Nosotros, Nosotras (f) = We
Novecientos = Ninety
Noventa = Ninety
noviembre = November
Nuera = Daughter-in-law
Nuestro (-os), Nuestra (-as) = Our
Nueve = Nine

Número de apartamento = Apartment number
Número de licencia = Driver's license number
Número de ochocientos = Eight hundred number
Número de seguro social = Social security number
Número de teléfono = Telephone number
Número de teléfono de su casa = Home telephone number
Número de teléfono de su empleo = Work telephone number

O

Observar = To observe
Ochenta = Eighty
Ocho = Eight
Ochocientos = Eight hundred
octubre = October
Ocupación = Occupation
Oeste = West
Oído = Inner ear
Ojo = Eye
Olvidar = To forget
Once = Eleven
Oprima este número. = Press this number.
Oreja = Ear
Orina = Urine
Orina con frecuencia = Frequent urination
Oro = Gold
Orofaringe = Oropharynx
Orzuelo = Stye
Oscuro = Dark

P

Paciente = Patient
Paciente externo = Out-patient
Paciente interno = In-patient
Padrastro = Step father
Padre = Father
Pagar = To pay
Paladar blando = Soft palate
Paladar duro = Hard palate
Palpitaciones = Arrhythmias
Páncreas = Pancreas
Paperas = Mumps

Para uso externo = For external use
Paramédico = Paramedic
Parche = Patch
Pare = Stop
Párpado = Eyelid
Pasillo = Aisle
Pastilla = Tablet, Lozenge
Pastillas para la tos = Cough drop
Pecho = Chest
Pediátrico = Pediatrics
Pene = Penis
Penicilina = Penicillin
Pequeño = Little
Pérdida súbita de peso = Sudden weight loss
Perdón = Excuse me.
Pestaña = Eyelash
Picazón = Itching
Pida este número. = Ask for this number.
Pie = Foot
Piel = Skin
Pierna = Leg
Píldora = Pill
Piojos = Lice
Plata = Silver
Poco = Sparingly
Policía = Police
Póngalo allí = Put it there
Por # días = For # days
Por # meses = For # months
Por # semanas = For # weeks
Por boca = By mouth
Por favor = Please
Por la mañana = In the morning
Por la noche = In the evening
Por la tarde = In the afternoon
Por qué = Why
Portero (a) = Janitor
Preguntar = To ask
Preparar = To prepare
Presión alta = High blood pressure
Presión arterial Presión sanguínea, Tensión arterial = Blood pressure
Prevenir = To prevent
Primer nombre = First name
Primo (m), Prima (f) = Cousin
Problemas sexuales = Sexual problems
Protección = Protection
Psoriasis = Psoriasis
Puede llamar más tarde = Could you call later
Puedo hablar con = May I speak to

Puedo servirle = May I help you
Pulmonía, Neumonía = Pneumonia
Pupila = Pupil
Qué = What

Q

Qué bonito *(m)* = How pretty
Qué hora es = What time is it
Qué le vaya bien, Tenga un buen día. = Have a nice day
Qué pasa = What's happening
Qué sonrisa = What a smile
Qué tiempo hace = What's the weather
Quejona = Ketone
Quemadura = Burn
Quetoacidosis = Ketoacidosis
Quién = Who
Quimioterapia = Chemotherapy
Quince = Fifteen
Quinientos = Five hundred
Quiste = Cyst
Quite estos = Remove these
Quizás = Maybe

R

Radiología = Radiology
Radioteléfono portátil = Two-way radio
Rayos equis = X-ray
Razón = Right
Recepcionista = Receptionist
Receta médica = Prescription
Recoja todo esto = Pick up all these
Recto = Rectum
Refrigerador = Refrigerator
Regresar = To return
Regrese pronto. = Come back soon.
Repita, por favor. = Repeat, please.
Resistencia = Resistance
Respiración corta = Shortness of breath
Retención de flujo = Fluid retention
Riesgo = Risk
Riesgo = Risk
Rociada = Spray
Rodilla = Knee
Rojo = Red
Rosa = Pink

S

sábado = Saturday
Sala de emergencia = Emergency room
Sala de espera = Waiting room

Sala de operaciones = Operating room
Sala de recuperación = Recovery room
Salida = Exit
Salina = Saline
Salón = Lobby
Sangrado = Bleeding
Sangre = Blood
Sanitarios, Baño = Rest rooms
Sarampión = Measles
Se puede repetir esta receta médica # veces. = You may repeat this prescription # times.
Se puede repetir esta una vez. = You may repeat this once.
Secretaria = Secretary
Sed = Thirsty
Sedante = Sedative
Según las instrucciones de su doctor. = As directed by your doctor
Segundo nombre = Middle name
Seis = Six
Seiscientos = Six hundred
Semen = Semen
Sensibilidad a la luz solar = Photosensitivity
Señor = Sir or Mister
Señora = Mrs. or Ma'am
Señorita = Miss
Separado *(a)* = Separated
septiembre = September
Sesenta = Sixty
Setecientos = Seven hundred
Setenta = Seventy
Sexo = Sex
Sexo oral = Oral sex
SIDA, Síndrome de inmunodeficiencia adquirida = AIDS
Siete = Seven
Sin protección = Without protection
Síndrome premenstrual = PMS
Síntomas = Symptoms
Sistema inmunitario = Immune system
Sobrepeso = Overweight
Sobrina = Niece
Sobrino = Nephew
Solo cuando es necesario = Only when necessary
Solo cuando tiene dolor = Only when you have pain
Soltero *(a)* = Single
Solución = Solution
Sótano = Basement

Su cuenta está # dólares. = Your total is # dollars.

Su doctor se cambió su receta médica. = Your doctor changed your prescription.

Su nombre, por favor = Your name, please

Su número, por favor = Your number, please

Su receta médica estará lista esta tarde. = Your prescription will be ready this afternoon.

Su receta médica estará lista mañana = Your prescription will be ready tomorrow

Su, Sus = His, her or Your (polite)

Sudores = Sweats

Suegra = Mother-in-law

Suegro = Father-in-law

Sueño = Sleepy

Supervisor *(a)* = Supervisor

Suplemento nutricional = Nutritional Supplement

Supositorio = Suppository

Supositorio rectal = Rectal Suppository

Supositorio vaginal = Vaginal Suppository

Sur = South

Susurro = Swish

T

Tableta, Pastilla = Tablet

Tapón de seguridad = Safety cap

Teléfono = Telephone

Teléfono celular = Cellular phone

Temblor = Tremor

Tendón = Tendon

Tengo el número equivocado. = I have the wrong number.

Terapeuta = Therapist

Terapia = Therapy

Terapia física = Physical therapy

Terapia respiratoria = Respiratory therapy

Tía = Aunt

Tienda de regalos = Gift shop

Tiene dolor = Do you have pain

Tiene dolor constante = Is the pain constant

Tiene dolor intermitente = Is the pain intermittent

Tiene dolor moderado = Is the pain mild

Tiene dolor muy fuerte = Is the pain severe

Tiene dolor profundo = Is the pain deep

Tiene dolor pulsante = Is the pain throbbing

Tiene dolor quemante = Is the pain burning

Tiene el número equivocado = You have the wrong number

Tiene mucho dolor = Do you have a lot of pain

Tiene seguro para su medicina = Do you have insurance for your medication

Tímpano = Ear drum

Tío = Uncle

Tipo dos = Type 2

Tipo uno = Type 1

Tobillo = Ankle

Tobillo = Ankle

Toma = Take

Toma _____ veces = Take _____ times

Toma dos tabletas por boca hoy = Take 2 tablets by mouth today

Toma la medicina = Take the medicine

Toma la medicina # veces por día. = Take the medicine # times per day.

Tomar = To take

Torcedura = Sprain

Tos = Cough

Trabajar = To work

Traiga = Swallow

Tráigame eso. = Bring me that

Tranquilizantes = Tranquilizers

Transmisión = Transmission

Trece = Thirteen

Treinta = Thirty

Tres = Three

Trescientos = Three hundred

Tu, Tus = Your

Tuberculosis = Tuberculosis

U

Úlcera = Ulcers

Un *(m)*, Una *(f)* = A or an

Un cuarto = One quarter

Un momento, por favor = One moment please

Un poco = A little

Un tercero = One third

Una media = Half

Uno = One

Unos, Unas = Some *(pl)*

Uña = Nail
Urticaria = Hives
Usa medicinas sin receta médica = Are you using over the counter medications
Usa productos naturales o remedios caseros = Are you using herbal products
Usa remedios caseros = Are you using home remedies
Usando los números de uno hasta diez, indique el nivel de su dolor = Using the numbers from one through ten indicate the level of your pain.
Usar = To use
Use para = Use for
Usted = You *(Polite)*
Ustedes = You *(Pl)*
Úvula = Uvula

V

Vacuna = Vaccine
Vagina = Vagina
Vámonos = Let's go
Varicela = Chicken pox
Vaso = Glass
Vaya con él = Go with him
Veces al día = Times per day
Veinte = Twenty
Veinte y cinco = Twenty five
Veinte y cuatro = Twenty four
Veinte y dos = Twenty two
Veinte y nueve = Twenty nine
Veinte y ocho = Twenty eight
Veinte y seis = Twenty six
Veinte y siete = Twenty seven
Veinte y tres = Twenty three
Veinte y uno = Twenty one
Venga aquí = Come here
Verde = Green
Vergüenza = Ashamed
Verificar = To verify
Vial = Vial
viernes = Friday
VIH, Virus de la inmunodeficiencia humana = HIV
Virus = Virus
Visión borrosa = Blurred vision
Visitante = Visitor
Vitaminas = Vitamins
Viudo *(a)* = Widow
Vomitando = Vomiting
Voy a buscar un traductor = I'm going to look for a translator

Voy a llamar a su doctor = I am going to call your doctor
Voy a llamar a su doctor para que autorice la repetición de esta receta médica = I am going to call your doctor for authorization to renew this prescription.

X

xx años = xx years old

Y

Ya me voy = I'm leaving now
Yerno = Son-in-law
Yo = I
Yo también = Me too
Yo tampoco = Me neither

Other Books in the SpeakEasy Spanish™ Series
Order Online at www.SpeakEasySpanish.com

Survival Spanish for All Americans
Survival Spanish for Apartment Managers
Survival Spanish for Churches and Mission Trips
Survival Spanish for Construction
Survival Spanish for Customer Service
Survival Spanish for Employers
Survival Spanish for Educators
Survival Spanish for First Responders
Survival Spanish for Healthcare
Survival Spanish for Legal Professionals
Survival Spanish for Pharmacists
Survival Spanish for Realtors
Survival Spanish for Restaurants and Hotels
Survival Spanish for Social Services

The SpeakEasy Spanish™ Audio Series
CD With Pronunciation Guide

Survival Spanish for All Americans
Survival Spanish for Apartment Managers
Survival Spanish for Construction
Survival Spanish for Pharmacists
Survival Spanish for Social Services

Invite Myelita to Speak at Your Next Event!

To inquire about cost and availability write to:
info@SpeakEasySpanish.com

Follow Myelita on Twitter and become a fan of SpeakEasy Spanish™ on Facebook

CPSIA information can be obtained
at www.ICGtesting.com
Printed in the USA
LVOW03s0052280616

494331LV00001B/1/P